Yana Nashua

Native American Herbalist's Bible

A Modern Guide To Native American Traditions and Customs. Everything You Need To Know About Herbalism, Apothecary, And Recipes To Naturally Improve Your Wellness

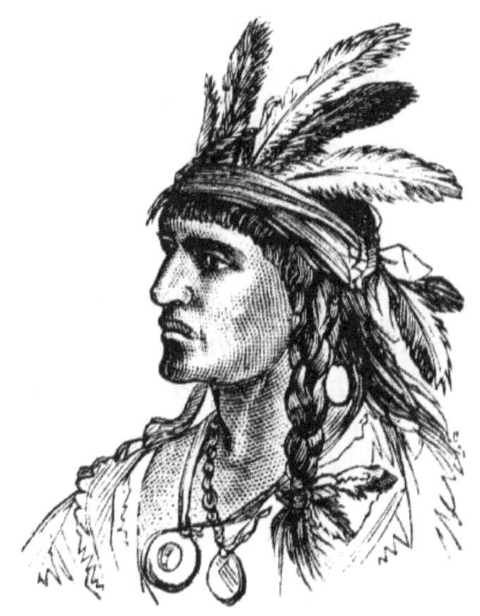

© Copyright 2021 by **Yana Nashua**

1

Table of Contents

Book 1

Native American spiritual history

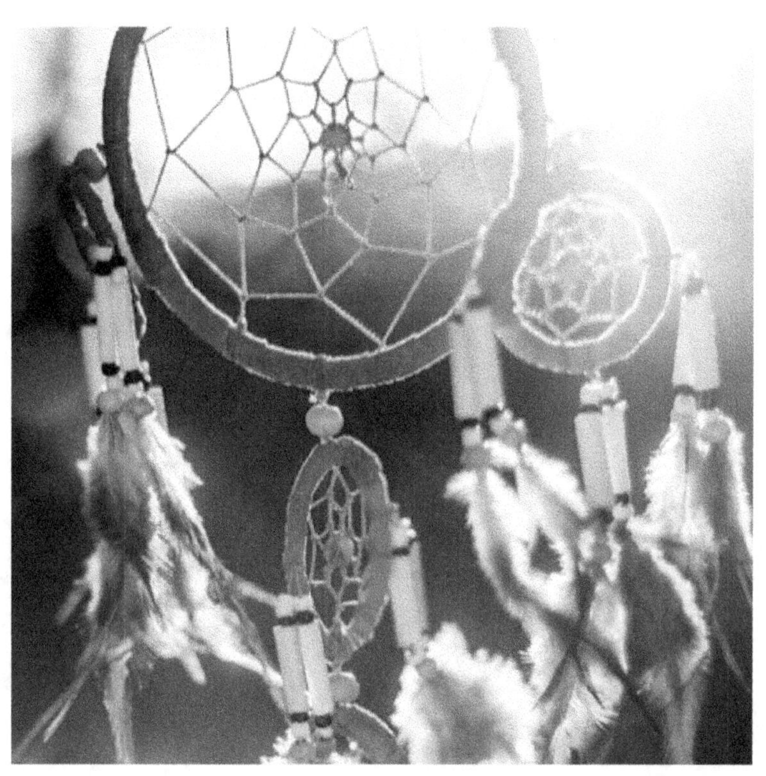

Introduction

American Indians: who they are, customs and traditions

Who are the ancient inhabitants of the "New Continent" really? The ancestors of Native Americans arrived in what is now the United States at least 15,000 years ago, perhaps much earlier, from Asia across the Bering Strait, developing a wide variety of peoples, societies, and cultures.

The European colonization of the Americas, which began in 1492, caused a rapid decline in the Native American population due to new diseases to which they had no immunity, ethnic cleansing, and slavery.

After its formation, the United States, as part of its colonial policy, continued to perpetrate massacres against many Native American peoples, dispossessed from their ancestral lands, and subjected to unilateral treaties and discriminatory government policies.

Today there are 574 federally recognized tribes living in the United States, about half of which are associated with Indian reservations.

American Indian customs

American Indians are generally known for having the spirit of warriors, being good hunters and having a great respect for nature. However, their customs and languages are very different among the various tribes.

It is estimated that when Europeans arrived in North America, there were more than 300 different indigenous languages among the tribes. Of these, more than half have disappeared and some of those that have survived are at risk of extinction.

One of the most popular American Indian customs are group dances, rituals that are performed for a variety of purposes, primarily to ask Mother

Nature for prosperity. Dances include the bison dance, the rain dance or the famous sun dance, propitiatory for the health of the tribe. Tribal leaders directed religious life and performed various rituals and ceremonies, some of which included fasting and offerings.

Another of the most important customs is pow-wow, or the gathering of the native tribes of North America, which is still held today.

Like their customs, each tribe's clothing was different. In general, men wore breeches and protected themselves from the cold with pants and deer and bison skin. For their part, women tended to wear leather dresses and foot-length robes. For ceremonial acts, some tribes wore special tunics decorated with feathers, animal skins and many other accessories and decorations.

American Indians: religions and beliefs

Native American religion and spiritual beliefs played an important role in their daily lives. Each tribe and people had its own unique belief system, legends, and rituals, all of which shared a great deal of animism.

Native Americans of the Pacific Northwest believed that all living things were guarded by guardian spirits. This included animals, trees, people, and even some inanimate objects such as wind, storms, and water. The Great Spirit was a supreme being who watched over everything, including the other spirits of the world. He could take different forms depending on the tribe: the Blackfoot people believed in the "Old Man", the creator of all things and the origin of spiritual wisdom.

Some Indian tribes in the southeaster United States believed in the "three worlds" including the upper world, the lower world and this world. The upper world was considered perfect and pure. The lower world was frightening and chaotic. Between the two was this world in which man lived. Spirits were able to travel between the different worlds and man was responsible for maintaining the balance between the three worlds.

In order to get closer to the spirits, some men would try to get hallucinations by taking drugs, fasting, being alone in the desert, or inflicting wounds on their bodies. Eventually, they hoped to get a vision from the spirits that would guide them or help them make an important life decision.

Yana Nashua

Religion in the life of Native Americans

The theme of religion pervades all studies of Indian culture. The Indians were a particularly pious and devout people, who considered themselves an extension of animate and inanimate nature. Religion and ritual were therefore a function of any activity: the search for food and other modes of survival, technology, social and political organization, warfare and art. Religion and magic were connected with practical science, as prayer was used in conjunction with the techniques of hunting and fishing, and spells accompanied herbal remedies to cure disease. For Indians, natural phenomena were inseparable from supernatural ones.

Myth was a way of understanding reality. Religion had an important role in the interpretation of the universe and in the adaptation of human activity to the surrounding nature.

In addition to the sense of the sacred, other considerations can also be made about Indian religion. Part of their very intimate relationship with nature is a sense of kinship with the natural world and the attribution of innate souls and human properties to plants, animals, inanimate objects, and natural phenomena. Indian religion usually involved the belief that the universe was full of supernatural forces and powerful spirits.

Shamanism was a common form of religious practice in which individuals sought to control those spirits through the use of magic. Other characteristics of many Indian cultures included a wealth of myths and legends, ceremonies and sacred objects, the pursuit of visions and the use of psychotropic plants to facilitate those visions, music and dance as part of the ritual, and the concept of sacrifice to gain the spirits' favor.

In addition to those common traits, Indian religion has an admirable variety of beliefs, sacred symbols, and religious systems. Different tribes or related groups of peoples had different views of the supernatural world, with varied types of deities and spirits: monotheistic, all-powerful, universal spirits such as the Manitou of the Algonquins, the Orenda of the Iroquois, and the Wakenda of the Sioux who are the source of all other spirits; pantheistic deities with specific images and attributes such as the Quetzalcoatl of Mexico, the Plumed Serpent, spectres or spirits of monsters, the spirits of natural phenomena such as the sun and rain gods, benevolent and guarding spirits such as the Katchina of the Hopi, and evil ones such as the Wendigo of the Algonquins.

Along with those different types of supernatural beings, Indian peoples had different mythologies and traditions regarding the creation and structure of the universe, a variety of myths, ceremonies, and sacred objects, and different systems of religious organization.

Some tribes had individual shamans or witch doctors, others had secret societies or witch doctors, and still others had priests.

To better clarify the difficult subject of Indian religion, in this chapter we aim to discuss the two major cultural currents, the tradition of hunting in the north and the tradition of agriculture in the south, which foreshadowed the great religious diversity at the time of the arrival of the white man, as well as the religious movements that arose as a reaction to the white man.

Religious evolution before "contact"

Native American religious beliefs, rituals, and myths appear to derive from the intertribal spread and exchange of two distinct cultural traditions. The oldest of these - the northern hunting tradition - dates back to the first arrival of Paleo Siberian peoples in North America during the Ice Age. Their ideology and forms of veneration were rooted in the ancient Palaeolithic way of life. Hunting and healing rituals and magic, the visionary ecstatic states of shamans, and the veneration of an animal god who protects game and regulates hunting are the hallmarks of the Northern hunting tradition. Perhaps the purest historical expression of this tradition were the ceremonies around the polar bear, in which the bear was immolated and then consumed in a communal meal, where the kinship between humans and the bear, god of the mountains, was commemorated. Such practices of bear veneration existed throughout the land along the Arctic Circle, from the reindeer-breeding Lapps to Scandinavia and across Siberia to the Ainu of northern Japan and the Eskimos and Algonquins of the northern latitudes of North America.

When the ancient Palaeolithic beliefs and rituals spread south, they mingled with the younger southern agrarian tradition that was expanding northward with the spread of corn from the valley of Mexico. In that second tradition secret priests and cults replaced the individualistic shamans of the northern hunting tradition as the religious leaders of society, and magic and hunting rituals were integrated into agrarian ceremonies devoted to the seasonal cycle of fruits to be harvested. Sacred stories of the Grain Mother, found in agrarian societies, interpreted ancient Animal Masters myths yet again, thus shifting the source of fertility and new life into plants.

In many North American corn-growing tribes, vestiges of an older hunting culture persisted alongside the planting, fertility, and harvest rituals of the younger Southern agrarian tradition. Vision-seeking by Plains tribes and the sacred pipe, witch doctor sects, and dog immolation, characteristic of Plains and Woodland civilizations, all trace back to ancient shamanistic practices. Indeed, when the calendar of rituals was adapted to the life cycle of the corn, as in the case of the Iroquois and Hopi, winter remained the sacred season, as it was in the hunting traditions of the North, that of the dances (animal dances) and healing ceremonies.

On the other hand, religious practices merged with the agrarian traditions of the South that were also widespread in non-agrarian cultures.

The Kuksu cult and rites of personification with the gods, found in Northern California, the secret societies and masked dances of the Northwest Coast, shared elements with the priest societies in the South, distinguished by their hierarchical system and esoteric veneration.

Religious resistance after the "contact"

During the conquest of indigenous America, Europeans waged war by both ideological and military and economic means against the integrity of indigenous American culture.

The European powers that colonized North America brought with them not only armies and merchants, but also missionaries to convert the Indians from their so-called "pagan" and "primitive" customs to the Christian religion and European customs. The resulting effect of Christianization was truly profound as were the Indian wars, the fur trade, and European diseases.

In cases where Spanish, French or English missionaries succeeded in Christianizing the Indians, the tribes disappeared as distinct political entities and cultures, their members absorbed into the dominant white man's culture and placed, usually, at the bottom of the social ladder, as in the case of the California Mission Indians who lived a serf-like existence in the Spanish feudal system. In some cases, however, attempts to Christianize the indigenous population met with stubborn resistance. The Pueblo rebellion of 1680 was one of the first revolts against foreign powers. Inspired by the doctrines of the prophet Pope, the rebels succeeded, albeit only briefly, in driving the Spanish out of New Mexico and re-establishing Indian religion and culture.

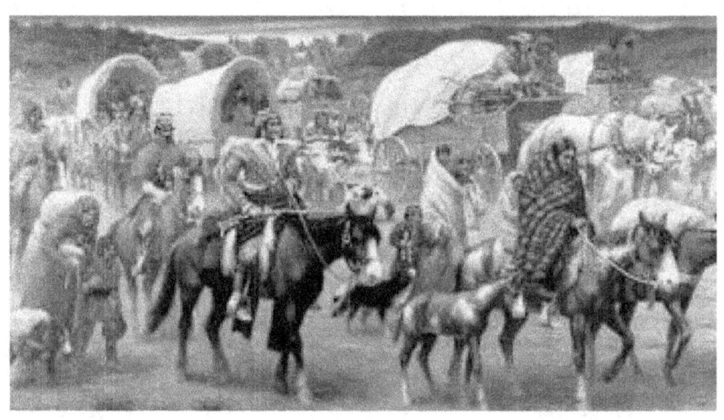

Later attempts to expel Europeans from North America manifested a similar pattern of prophethood and resistance. The Pontiac, Tecumseh, and Black Hawk intertribal movements in the second half of the eighteenth century and the first half of the nineteenth took their impetus from the doctrines of Delaware, Shawnee, and Winnebago prophets and Indian priests who preached resistance against white man culture and a return to pre-Contact ways of life.

The apocalyptic tone of those prophets suggests that they preached certain themes taken from Christianity itself, especially the appeal to the Old Testament prophets, in order to purify the people from outside influences and, with suffering, prepare for a revival of Indian religion and culture.

Other currents of Indian religious renewal, often with Christian elements, occurred during the same period. In 1799 Handsome Lake founded the "Longhouse" religion among the Iroquois, which not only reaffirmed the validity of Iroquois beliefs, but also adapted them to the realities of military defeat and cultural subjugation, offering the Indians a way to move from the ancient tribal system of communal property held in clan hands to a new form of family farm and private property.

Many revival movements followed during the latter part of the nineteenth century, on the plains and in the Far-West, due to military defeat and the disappearance of the buffalo. The religious movements of Smohalla and his dreamers, of John Slocum's "Indian Shaker Church" and of Wovoka's "Ghost Dance Religion" developed equally in an apocalyptic direction. The "Ghost

Dance" religion, which spread from tribe to tribe, culminated at Wounded Knee in 1890, where Wovoka's prophecy about the return of slain warriors and buffaloes to chase away the white man met the cruel reality of American guns in a massacre that the magical armored shirts of the "Ghost Dancers" could certainly not prevent.

At the turn of the twentieth century the last great Indian prophet, Quanah Parker, discovered the Peyote Road and helped found the Native American Church which spread among the defeated peoples of the Southeast, Plains, Prairies, Great Lakes and urban areas. Offering a liturgy and sacrament of Peyote, the Native American Church was a variant of Christian veneration in that it challenged some ancient beliefs and ceremonies.

The main Native American religions

Religion of the Earth Lodge

The Earth Lodge Religion was founded in Northern California and Southern Oregon tribes such as the Wintun . It spread to tribes such as Achomawi , Shasta and Siletz , just to name a few . It was also known as the "Warm House Dance". It predicted events similar to those predicted by the Ghost Dance, such as the return of the ancestors or the end of the world. The Religion of the Earth Lodge influenced the next religious practice, the Dream Dance, belonging to the Klamath and Modoc.

Ghost Dance

The Ghost Dance movement of the late 1800s was a religious revitalization movement in the western United States. Initially founded as a local ceremony in Nevada, by the Paiute prophet Wodziwob , the movement did not gain widespread popularity until 1889-1890, when the Ghost Dance Religion was founded by Wovoka (Jack Wilson), who was also Northern Paiute . The Ghost Dance was created in a time of genocide, to save the lives of Native Americans by enabling them to survive current and impending catastrophes, calling the dead to fight on their behalf, and to help them drive settlers from their lands.

In December 1888, Wovoka, thought to be the son of medicine man Tavibo (Numu-tibo'o), fell ill with a fever during a solar eclipse on January 1, 1889. After his recovery, he claimed to have visited the spirit world and the Supreme Being and predicted that the world would soon end, only to be restored to a pure state in the presence of the Messiah. All Native Americans would inherit this world, including those who had already died, to live eternally without suffering. To achieve this reality, Wovoka stated that all Native Americans should live honestly and avoid the ways of whites (especially alcohol consumption). He called for meditation, prayer, song, and dance as an alternative to mourning for the dead because they would soon be resurrected. Wovoka's followers saw it as a form of the messiah and it became known as the "Red Man Christ."

Tavibo had participated in the Ghost Dance of 1870 and had a similar vision of the Great Spirit of the Earth removing all white men, and then of an earthquake removing all humans. Tavibo's vision concluded that Native Americans would return to live in a restored environment and that only believers in his revelations would be resurrected.

This religion spread to many tribes on western reservations, including Shoshone , Arapaho , Cheyenne and Sioux (Dakota, Lakota and Nakota). In fact, some Lakota and Dakota bands were so desperate for hope during this period of forced relocation and genocide that, after making a pilgrimage to the Nevada Ghost Dance in 1889-1890, they became more militant in their resistance to white settlers. Each nation that adopted the Ghost Dance way provided its own understanding to the ceremony, which included predictions that whites would disappear, die, or be pushed back across the sea. A Ghost Dance rally at Wounded Knee in December 1890 was invaded by the Seventh

Cavalry, which massacred unarmed Lakota and Dakota, primarily women, children, and the elderly.

The early Ghost Dance heavily influenced religions such as Earth Lodge, Bole-Maru Religion, and Dream Dance. The Caddo Nation and many other communities still practice Ghost Dance today, though usually in secret.

Native Shaker Religion

Also known as Tschida, the Native Shaker Religion was influenced by the Waashat Religion and founded by John Slocum , a member of Squaxin Island. The name comes from the shaking and spasming movements used by participants to sweep away their sins. The religion combines Christianity with traditional Indian teachings. This religion is still practiced today in the Indian Shaker Church.

Longhouse Religion

The Longhouse Religion is the popular name of the religious movement known as The Code of Handsome Lake or Gaihwi: io ("Good Message"), founded in 1799 by the Seneca prophet Handsome Lake (Sganyodaiyo ?). This movement combines and reinterprets elements of traditional Iroquois religious beliefs with elements adopted from Christianity, primarily by Quakers. Gaihwi: io currently has about 5,000 practicing members. Originally Gaihwi: io was known as the "new religion" in opposition to the prevailing animistic beliefs, but has since become known as the "old religion" in opposition to Christianity.

Mexicayotl

Mexicayotl (Nahuatl word meaning "Essence of Mexico ", "Mexicanity"; Spanish : Mexicanidad ; see -yotl) is a movement reviving the indigenous religion , philosophy and traditions of ancient Mexico (Aztec religion and Aztec philosophy) among the Mexican people.

The movement came to light in the 1950s, led by intellectuals in Mexico City , but has only grown significantly at the grassroots level in more recent times, spreading to Chicanos in North America. Their rituals involve mitotiliztli. The followers, called Mexicatl (singular) and Mexicah (plural), or simply Mexica , are mostly urban and suburban people.

The Mexicayotl movement began in the 1950s with the founding of the group Nueva Mexicanidad by Antonio Velasco Piña . In the same years, Rodolfo Nieva López founded the "Movimiento Confederado Restaurador de la Cultura del Anáhuac", whose co-founder was Francisco Jimenez Sanchez who in the following decades became a spiritual leader of the Mexicayotl movement, endowed with the honorary title Tlacaelel . He had a profound influence in shaping the movement, founding the In Kaltonal ("House of the Sun," also called the Native Church of Mexico) in the 1970s.

From the 1970s onward Mexcayotl grew by developing into a network of local worship and community groups (called calpulli or kalpulli) and spreading to Mexican Americans or Chicanos in the United States . It has also developed strong ties to Mexican national identity movements and Chicano nationalism. The Native Mexican Church of Sanchez (which is a confederation of calpullis) was officially recognized by the government of Mexico in 2007.

Native American Church

The Peyote religion, legally called and more properly known as the Native American Church, has also been called the "Peyote Road" or "Peyote Way," is a religious tradition involving the ceremonial and sacred use of *Lophophora williamsii* (peyote). The use of peyote for religious purposes is thousands of years old and some have thought it originated within one of the following tribes: the Carrizo, the Lipan Apache , the Mescalero Apache , the Tonkawa, the Karankawa or the Caddo , with the Cree Plains, Carrizo and Lipan Apache being the three most likely sources. In Mexico the Huichol, Tepehuan, and other native Mexicans use peyote. Since then, despite numerous efforts to make peyote ceremonies illegal, the ceremonial use of peyote has spread from the area of Mexico to Oklahoma and other western parts of the United States. Notable members of the Native American Church (NAC) include Quannah Parker , the founder of NAC, and Big Moon of the Kiowa tribe.

Waashat Religion

The Waashat religion is also called the Washani Religion, Longhouse Religion, Religion of the Seven Drums, Sunday Dance Religion, Prophet's Dance, and Faith of the Dreamers. The Indian Wanapam Smohalla (c. 1815-1895) used wáashat rituals to build the religion in the Pacific Northwest . Smohalla claimed that visions came to him through dreams and that he had visited the spirit world and been sent back to teach his people. The name waasani spoke of what the religion was about; it meant both dance and worship. He led a return to the original way of life before white influences and established ceremonial music and dances. Smohalla's speech was called Yuyunipitqana for "Screaming Mountain."

The Faith of the Dreamers, and its dance elements, foreshadowed the later Ghost Dances of the peoples of the plains. It was a religion of return to our heritage. Believers believed that whites would disappear and nature would return as it was before they came. In order to achieve this, the natives must do the things required by the spirits, like a Weyekin. What the spirits wanted was to get rid of violent ways, get rid of white culture, and not buy, sell, or disrespect the Earth. They must also dance the Dance of the Prophet (wáashat).

The religion combined elements of Christianity with Native beliefs, but rejected white American culture. This made it difficult for the United States to assimilate or control the tribes. The United States was trying to convert the Plains tribes from hunter-gatherers to farmers, in the European-American tradition. They wanted to remake the Natives, but found a problem with those who followed the Dreamer Cult: "Their model of a man is an Indian; they aspire to be an Indian and nothing else."

Prophets of the movement included Smohalla (of the Wanapam people), Kotiakan (of the Yakama nation), and Homli (of the Walla Walla). Their messages were carried down the Columbia River to other communities. It is unclear exactly how it began or when Christianity influenced the earlier form, but it is thought to have something to do with the arrival of non-Indians or an epidemic and a prophet with an apocalyptic vision. The Waashat dance involves seven drummers, a salmon feast, the use of eagle and swan feathers, and a sacred song sung every seventh day.

Cruzo'ob Maya

Cruzo'ob is the name by which a group of Yucatec Maya rebels were designated during the Caste War that took place in the Yucatan Peninsula from 1847 to 1901. The term is composed of the word cross in the Spanish language and 'ob from the Mayan language. The Caste War started by a social movement in 1847, three years later, took a religious turn with the appearance of the Mayan Cross (Talking Cross). According to legend, the cult of the Cross is attributed to the soldier José María Barrera, Manuel Nahuat and Juan de la Cruz Puc. Barrera left the ranks of the Yucatan government to join the Mayan rebels. In 1850 according to the White Yucatecos, near a cenote, Barrera formed three crosses in a tree, with the help of Manuel Nahuat, a Mayan with ventriloquist skills, managed to convince his companions of the discovery of a "holy cross". In the version of the Mayan legend, the Cross appeared near a cenote and inspired the Mayans to continue fighting. On October 15, 1850 appears the proclamation of Juan de la Cruz Puc, Mayan leader and interpreter of the cross. The Holy Cross Maya is the supreme symbol of the rebellious Maya Yucateca and Juan is seen as a prophet. Juan de la Cruz Puc's sermons and prophecies are collected in the A'almaj T'aan, which is considered the Bible among the Cruzo'ob faith. The rebellious Maya believed that through the cross, God communicated with them. In this way, the city of Noh Cah Santa Cruz Balam Nah Kampocolché Cah was founded and the cult of the Holy Cross (Talking Cross), the place became the capital of the Mayan state known as Chan Santa Cruz (Little Holy Cross).

On March 23, 1851, the community was attacked by the Yucateco army under the orders of Colonel Novelo, during the siege Manuel Nahuat died, and the colonel took the three crosses. José María Barrera survived the attack, established again the cult of the Cross, which, from then on, communicated with the Maya only in writing. Barrera died at the end of 1852, but the cult was preserved and the followers of the Cross became known as cruzo'ob. The rebels were organized into a military theocracy similar to pre-Hispanic models. The top leader was the Tata Chikiuc, the political-religious leader was the Nohoch Tata, and the keeper of the cross was the Tata Polin. In contrast, whites were known as dzulob (dzul singular). The Cruzo'ob faith began as a syncretic religion between Christianity and Mayan spirituality. The faith is primarily practiced in the Mexican state of Quintana Roo and to a lesser extent in northern Belize.

Stomp Dance

The walking dance, called sayvtketv by the Muscogee Creek, hilha by the Chickasaw and Choctaw and gatiyo alisgisdi by the Cherokee, is a religious/social tradition celebrated by some indigenous peoples of the southeastern woods. Those who are known to celebrate it, or have celebrated it previously, are Muscogee Creek, Alabama, Koasati, Coosa, Coweta, Taskigi,

Yamasee, Okfuski, Yuchi, Chiaha, Kasihta, Okmulgi, Seminole, Chickasaw, Choctaw, Cherokee, Hainai, Nabedache, Nabiti, Nacogdoche, Nacono, Nadaco, Nasoni, Nechaui, Neche, Kadohadacho, Nanatsoho, Doustioni, Adai, Cahinnio, Eyeish, Ouachita, Tula, Yatasi, Natchez, Peoria, Miami, Shawnee, Ottawa, Delaware, Tuscarora, Houma, Chakchiuma, Seneca-Cayuga, as well as many others who belonged to the Mississippian Sphere of ideological interaction.

The stomping dance, if ceremonial, is usually held in a designated dance field, but can be held anywhere if it is social. It may be preceded by the game of stickball, a game that was previously surrounded by much ceremonial practice. When the sun goes down, men gather in arbores, the amount of which depends on the tribe. Women and children sit around the ceremonial square next to the arbores. The chief's speaker will call out who will lead the first song and ask all the men to say "hoo" and step up. Then all the men will call the women forward, calling them "turtles," due to the fact that they shake the shells on their legs. After this, the women come forward and they all dance various dances throughout the night, such as the snake dance, friendship dance, ribbon dance, etc. Participants will "touch medicine" throughout the night, which is meant to give participants purification and strength.

Participants will often eat traditional foods during the gathering. Foods such as hominy, cornbread, pashofa, lye/grape dumplings, salt meat, fried bread, wild onions/ramps and three sisters' vegetables are usually eaten during the dances. Community is very important in tribes as it preserves teachings and practices that could be lost without it. Stomp dance is just one of those ways that tribes communicate with each other.

Yana Nashua

The socio-political organization of Native Americans

For most indigenous North Americans, as indeed for most peoples throughout human history, there were no institutionalized forms of social and political power, no state, no bureaucracy, and no army. American Indian societies were as a rule egalitarian without a central authority and social hierarchy, typical of modern societies. Customs and traditions instead of law and coercion governed social life.

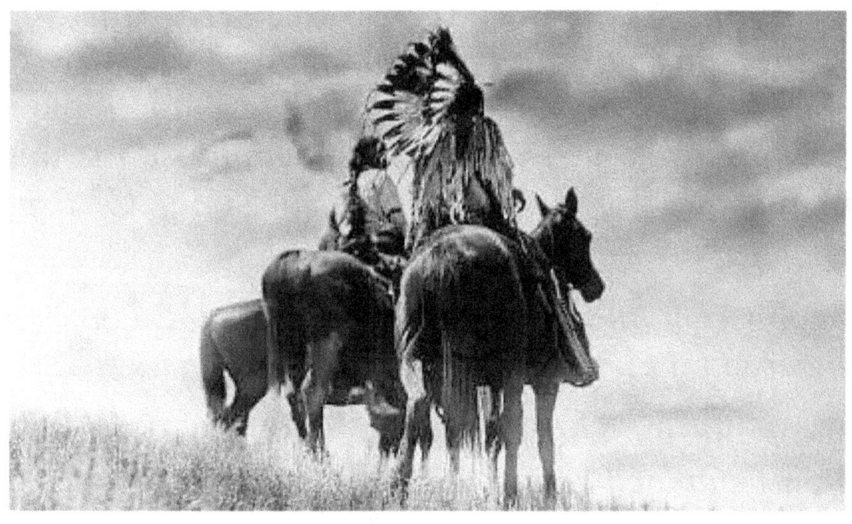

Where chiefs existed, their influence was usually based on personal qualities and not on formal or permanent status. One of the earliest French missionaries, to the Montagnais-Naskapi, Labrador Indians, Father Le Jeune, observed in 1634 that "the Indians would not stand at all for those who wish to assume superiority over others." Authority within a group derived from the ability to make useful proposals and knowledge of tribal tradition and folklore.

Among the Eskimos, for example, an important person was called Isumatag meaning "the one who thinks."

Anthropologists have invented various socio-political classification systems for different peoples in North America. More than 20 years ago Elman Service found that Indian societies at the time of white contact exhibited a wide range of evolving types, from simple groupings of tribes and tribal leaders, to the highly organized state of the Aztecs in the valley of Mexico. Although Service's scheme has been questioned and revised by others, it offers a comparative perspective concerning the socio-political organization of indigenous cultures, where an institutionalized central supremacy is manifested that defines a continuity from the simplest egalitarian societies to the most complex and most stratified.

Grouping was the typical form of social organization of hunters and gatherers, such as the Eskimos of the Arctic areas, the Algonquins and Atapascans of the Subarctic and the Shoshoni of the Great Basin. Those peoples lived in harsh environments that could only support low density populations. Groupings (bands) were isolated family units and some might seasonally join together for collective hunting, only to disperse again to different hunting grounds.

Political leadership remained informal and personal. Cooperation between families was ensured by kinship and marriage alliances.

Kinship is one of the most difficult and most debated aspects of Indian culture, as systems changed and created confusion.

Given the complexity and controversy surrounding it, the topic is touched on only briefly: kinship - on this anthropologists seem to agree - was a social bond of cooperation and non-violence, a means of maintaining political alliances and economic relations in societies without order and laws. Kinship also regulated the social position of the individual. Kinship ties determined the line of descent, which could be patrilineal (through men only), matrilineal (through women only), or through women and men. Individual lineage is often part of a larger system of intermarital lineages that decide the possible spouse and in some cases the place of residence; that is, whether the wife lives with her husband's family (patrilocal) or whether the husband lives with his wife's (madrilocal).

Individual lineage is, as a rule, among Indians, exogamic, that is, the individual marries outside his lineage, as opposed to endogamic lineage, where the individual must marry within his family, clan, or social class.

Among the simplest societies, for example the Shoshoni, kinship ties were not emphasized and only the taboo of incest served as a rule for marriages. Among other groupings, such as the Algonquins and Atapascans, there was a tendency to formalize the relationship between cooperating families and to establish fixed rules regarding marriage and residence. The Serrano of Southern California, were an example of hunters and gatherers who had a complex kinship system, including patrilocal kinship, tracing lineages in the male line to a common ancestor and a middle structure, dividing all lineages into two larger groups with intermarriage.

The tendency to formalize kinship relationships shifted to another level of organization in the case of societies that could be called tribal. With greater population density due to agriculture or abundant wild food resources, indigenous cultures faced the problem of establishing fixed, cohesive work groups for various seasonal tasks. The spontaneous division of labor in the natural family was being replaced in many such societies by kinship relationships and classification systems invented to ensure the continuity of social ties and economic cooperation. The clans of the northeaster and Great Plains tribes along with the Southwestern Pueblo descended from a common mythical ancestor or totemic animal; thus a system of interdependent lineages was created and related by marriage, whose reciprocal relationships made the tribes larger political entities. The principle adopted in this regard is set by anthropologists as "fission and fusion"; that is, when society is segmented into autonomous families, clans, or local settlements, potential political divisions within the tribe are overcome by cultural similarities of language and custom, of practices of exogamy and of marriage alliances, plus pan-tribal societies of priests, warriors, and artisans. While one society or clan could stand out, none or none was superior.

Even in cases where broader political and military alliances were established in the form of tubal confederations, such as the Iroquois League, there was no sovereign authority beyond the local group and leadership was vested in reputable chiefs or councils of elders.

Instead, the tribal system of the Northwest Coast and Southeast, was based on hierarchical societies where lineage and community groups were no longer equal in principle, but arranged hierarchically, with superior authority conferred on certain families. Authority was also centralized according to the rule of primogeniture: social position was inherited according to birth order, and the first child had the highest rank. Broader political authority allowed chiefs to carry out activities on a larger scale, for example military and commercial expeditions or the construction of irrigation systems and temples. The tribal chief was responsible for intensifying production, redistributing wealth, and

to support craftsmen in the manufacture of luxury goods for the conspicuous consumption of noble families.

Although the tribal chief's rank was based on a centralized political authority hardly imaginable in tribal societies, the chief's power was limited. The social systems with their tribal chiefs were in effect theocratic societies in which the common people submitted to the religious authority and aristocratic ethos of the priest-chief and the nobility; however, they were not instruments of authority in that the ruling class ruled by force and maintained a stable army. As for the next level of socio-political organization, the formation of an actual state in Mesoamerica, kings, like tribal leaders, were high priests of a regent theocracy that had demanded religious loyalty from the population. But they were also the leaders of a regent theocracy that controlled the political, legal, and military apparatuses and had the exclusive right to use force.

The Aztec theocracy and its noble warriors extended their power throughout Mesoamerica by waging war against other peoples and cultures, and demanding tribute. Tenochtitlan in the Valley of Mexico, whose wealth and splendour inspired awe in the Spaniards (who visited it during the time of Cortes and which Cortes himself called "the most beautiful city in the world"), was the Aztec center for culture and power. The city displayed a *metropolitan order, far removed from any egalitarian concept of tribal groupings and societies and far more specialized and stratified than tribal societies, with their leaders, including the highly organized Natchez society.*

Complex social ties replaced the ancient kinship relationships of traditional Indian culture, and the various classes of warriors, merchants, and artisans existed alongside that of the ruling nobility. Whether the pochteca, the Aztec merchant class, had gradually assumed power, as had happened in other societies of the world and, according to what some scholars speculate might have happened, is a very difficult question to clarify, since history has erased everything through the military conquest of the Spanish conquistadores.

Yana Nashua

The Native American Code of Ethics

We should learn a lot from the great Native American people to live harmoniously in peace and love .Here is their code of ethics that can teach us how to live.

It is very easy to live harmoniously with joy if only we want to, and to teach us this is a great people almost extinct by those who thought they knew better. Those who extinguished this people now live in greed, unhappiness and war, the Native Americans instead have been able to live harmoniously among themselves, in perfect symbiosis with nature, thanks to their code of ethics, which should be a lesson for all the peoples of the earth.

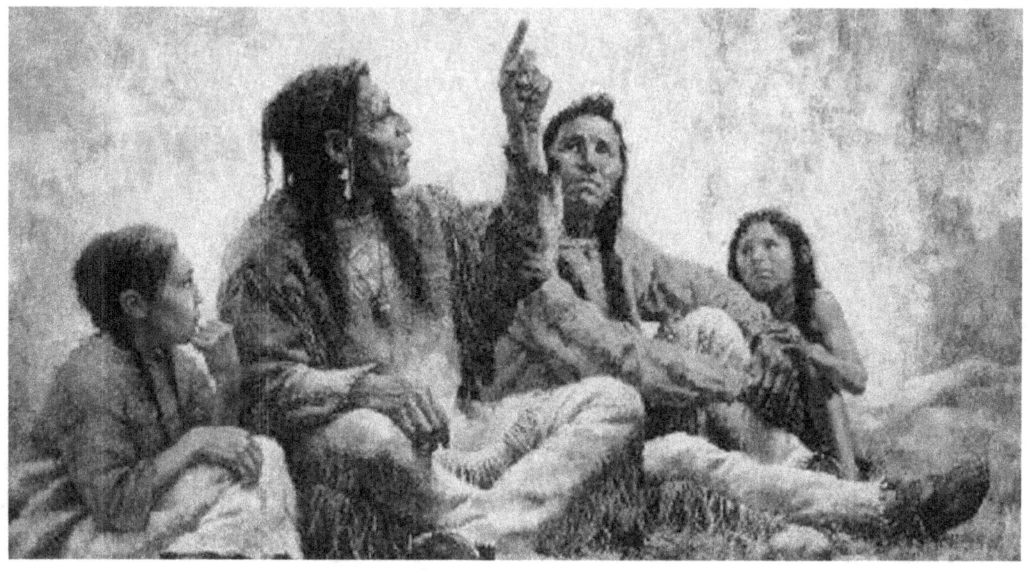

Native American culture is highly spiritual and places great emphasis on respecting Mother Earth, Father Sky, Grandfather Sun and Grandmother Moon as all living and non-living things.

The 20 most important rules of the Native American code of ethics

1. Pray alone. Pray often. The Great Spirit will hear you if only you speak.
2. Be tolerant of those who have lost their way. Ignorance, conceit, anger, jealousy and greed spring from a lost soul. Pray that they may find their way.
3. Seek yourself, be yourself. Don't allow others to create the path for you. It is your path and yours alone. Others can walk with you but no one can walk for you.
4. Treat guests in your home with great consideration. Serve them the best food and give them the best bed and treat them with respect and honour.
5. Do not take what is not yours, either from a person, a community, a desert or a culture. It has not been earned or given. It is not yours.
6. Respect everything on earth that is a person or plant.
7. Respect other people's thoughts, desires and words. Never interrupt another, mock them, or imitate them with derision.
8. Do not speak ill of others. The negative energy you put out into the universe will multiply when it comes back to you.
9. Everyone makes mistakes and all mistakes can be forgiven.
10. Bad thoughts cause diseases of the mind body and spirit. Practice optimism.
11. Nature is not for us but a part of us. It is part of your earthly family.
12. Children are the seeds of our future. Plant love in their hearts and water them with wisdom and life lessons. When they are grown give them room to grow.
13. Avoid hurting the hearts of others. The poison of your suffering will come back to you.
14. Always be honest. Honesty is proof of who you are in the universe.

15. *Stay balanced. Your mental, spiritual, emotional and physical selves, all of these parts need to be strong pure and healthy. Train your body and strengthen your mind. Grow rich in spirit to heal emotional afflictions.*

16. *Make conscious decisions about how you will be and react. Be responsible for your actions.*

17. *Respect the privacy and personal space of others. Do not touch others' personal property, especially sacred and religious property. This is forbidden.*

18. *Be true first and foremost to yourself. You cannot nurture and help others if you cannot first nurture and help yourself.*

19. *Respect other religious beliefs. Don't force your faith on others.*

20. *Share your good fortune with others. Be involved in charity.*

Yana Nashua

The Medicine Wheel

Medicine in the various languages and dialects of Native Americans has a very wide meaning that wants to symbolize all that is good, that has spirit, that has heart. Francis La Fleche, an ethnologist belonging to the Osage-Sioux tribe described the power, the "medicine" inherent in all things as follows: "Every living thing is wakan. Wakan is everything that possesses a power, whether it be active, like that of the wind or that which pushes the clouds, or passive, of resistance, of endurance, like that of the pebbles found along the roads. Even the most insignificant stick or stone has a particular spiritual essence that is imagined as a manifestation of that mysterious power that penetrates everything, that informs the entire universe of itself". Thus from the most ancient ages, the memory of which is hidden among the subtle plots of time, men sought to secure these powers, these formidable forces.

Indian Medicine Wheel

For the Indians of the prairies it was fundamental to look for their own guardian spirits, who could manifest themselves during a fast in the desert or during meditation on the top of a mountain; who could show themselves in sleep as in wakefulness, through a vision or even in the form of a natural event.

These "guardian spirits" provided their protégés with advice or instructed them in the manufacture of particularly potent "medicines".

According to the tradition of the American Indians, at the dawn of creation, since Wakan Tanka, the Great Spirit, put his hand to the creation of the universe, the earth was inhabited by other first-born beings, endowed with a dual nature: that of men and animals. After the advent of men, the second-born, these legendary beings, endowed with the ability to assume human form at will, retreated into the woods and waters, hidden where the eyes of no mortal could see them, in hidden places where only a few privileged men could visit them.

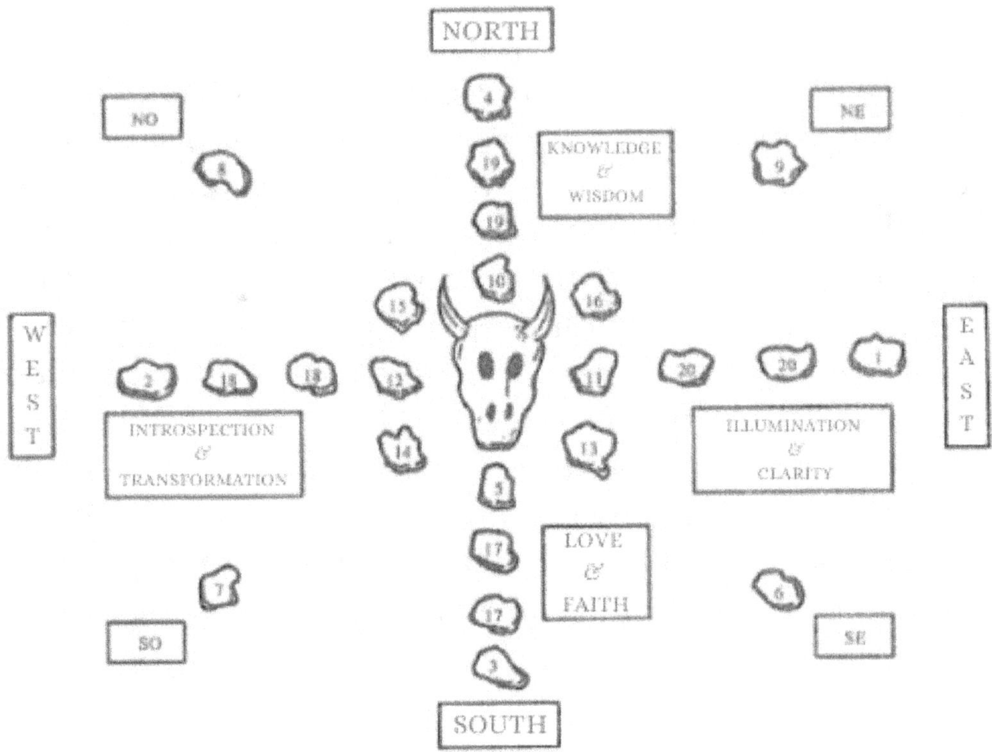

For the Indians of the Great Plains many were the sacred objects, among them drawings, songs, cosmic symbols, numbers, as well as the single components of "personal medicines". The most sacred of all things, however, the one that had a meaning of particular importance, was the sacred circle, manifestation of all cosmic forces, such as the Indian samsara or the Chinese tao. In this regard Black Elk is useful as always: "After the ceremony of the heyoka, I came to live here, where I am now, between the streams Wounded Knee and Grass. Others came with us, and we built these little gray log houses that you see, and they are square. It is a bad way to live, for there can be no power in a square. You have observed that everything an Indian does in is in a circle, and this is because the Power of the World always works in circles, and everything tries to be round. In days gone by, when we were a strong and happy people, all our power came to us from the sacred circle of the

nation, and until that circle was broken, the people flourished. The flourishing tree was the living center of the circle, and the circle of the four quadrants nourished it. The east gave peace and light, the south gave warmth, the west gave rain, and the north, with its cold and powerful wind, gave strength and endurance. This knowledge came to us from the world beyond, with our religion. Everything that the Power of the World does, it does in a circle. The sky is round, and I have heard that the earth is round like a ball, and so are the stars. The wind, when it is most powerful, turns in whirlwinds. The birds make their nests circular, for their religion is the same as ours. The sun always rises and sets in a circle. The moon does the same, and both are round. Even the seasons form a great circle, in their change, and always return to the point they were before. Man's life is a circle, from infancy to childhood, and the same happens with everything where a power moves. Our tents were round, like the nests of birds, and moreover they were always arranged in a circle, the circle of the nation, a nest of many nests, where the Great Spirit wanted us to brood our young. But the Wasichu put us in these square boxes. Our power is gone and we are dying, because the power is no longer in us. You can take a look at our kids and see how it is. When we were living by the power of the circle in the proper way, boys were becoming men at twelve, thirteen years old. But now they take a lot longer to mature. Patience, things are as they are. We are prisoners of war while we are down here waiting. But there's another world...".

The sacred circle and its power are therefore the fundamental assumptions on which the "medicine wheel" is also based, a sort of magic circle which, normally made of small stones or pebbles, contains all the principles of the universe and represents with them the infinite elements that compose it. Normally the wheel is divided into four quadrants (also subdivided), each of which wants to represent the four basic principles of which the universe is composed (respectively, starting from the south, water, earth, air and fire) as well as spirits, animals and cardinal points that are linked to these principles: the north, to which is associated the color white and from which "comes the great white wind that purifies", is the place where the giant Waziah lives; to the south is associated the color yellow and from it comes the summer and the power that makes it grow, here lives the White Swan who awaits the life of all peoples of the universe; to the west, where live the beings of thunder that send the rain and where the sun sets there is the color black: here dwells Wakinian-Tanka, the great Thunder Bird of the West, "in a hut on top of a mountain at the edge of the world where the sun sets"; to the east there is instead red, for here lives the "Morning Star" to give wisdom to men and its symbol is the eagle, Huntka, the animal that sees all. The center of the circle represents the sacred tree that joins the sky to the earth: it is "the tree of the world, whose trunk - which is also the column of the sun, the pole of sacrifice and the axis mundi - rising from the altar to the omphalos of the earth crosses the door of the world and branches above the roof of the world.

The day of the birth of each being is marked by a given position of this wheel: each one is therefore predisposed to the perception of the world according to the gifts received at that moment in function of the orientation of the wheel; the individual is in fact only a small part of an infinite cosmos and his task is the search of the balance of all that surrounds him, of the universal harmony: he is a small part of the wheel as the drop is of the sea. Just for the fact of being linked to a position of the wheel and with a particular animal or object, each Indian has a specific power and a specific position within his people, nation and all that surrounds him: just to this particular power they received and to the guardian spirit that belongs to them, Indians owe their name.

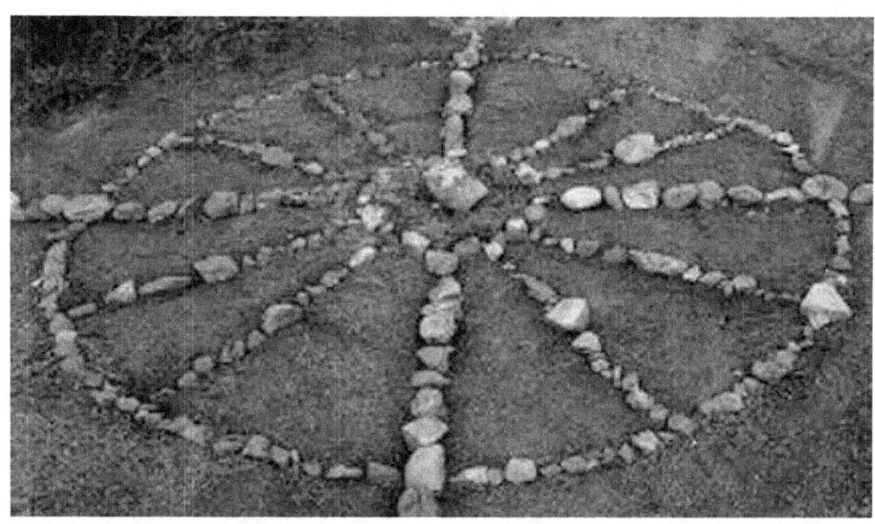

To particular men, endowed with great power, obtained after having returned from the world of the dead, is destined the performance of sacred ceremonies, healing and knowledge of the most sacred traditions: these are the wichasa wakan, the shamans, the medicine men: they are appointed to interpret visions, to receive the indications of the spirits, to treat herbs and to be the guardians of the sacred circle of the nation. The medicine wheel is thus an image, the means by which the power that binds all the things that make up the entire universe is channelled and that makes the whole sacred, that makes everything wakan.

Medicine Man and Spirits

The most interesting thing among the practices of the medicine man was the extraordinary ritual he used to get in touch with the spirits.

Whenever he wanted to foretell the future, to know the outcome of some future event or to cure some sick person at the point of death, he celebrated the ritual in the great tepee of medicine and the whole tribe could attend.

About an hour before the ceremony began, the herald went around the camp to announce that the medicine man was preparing to speak with the spirits.

The news caused great excitement.

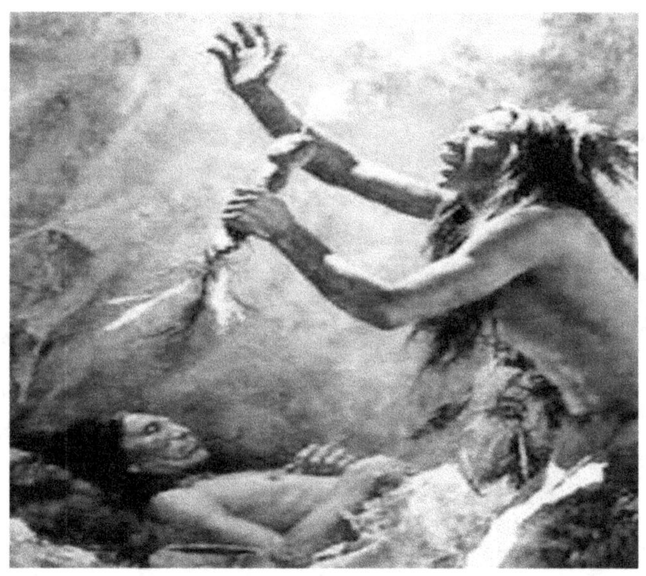

The members of the tribe went in time to the medicine hut to find a place, since only about one hundred people could enter, while the others had to stay outside, limiting themselves to follow with their ears the mysterious ceremony.

Here is what happened: the assistant of the medicine man planted 4 poles in the center of the shed, tying them together with crossed ends, so that under the poles was to form a clearing of about 4 meters wide and, in which the assistant, with the help of 4 men, planted a series of sharp pegs, placing them about 2 meters to about 2 cm and a half away from each other, to cover the entire area.

These pegs were so sharp that they would pierce the foot of any man who tried to walk on them.

In the center of the area a small gap was left, just enough for a man to stand upright.

The only way to reach it was to jump over the sharp pegs, and it was clear that you ran the risk of killing yourself or at least seriously injuring yourself.

The medical man then made his entrance accompanied by 4 assistants.

The 4 undressed him, leaving only his pants on and then they laid him on his back.

They joined his hands, palm to palm together and with a strong leather strap about bound his thumbs, so tight that sometimes the blood spurted.

And in the same way they joined and bound together each pair of fingers.

Then they would move on to the feet and join the two toes together, pulling with all their might to bind them as tightly as they could.

At this point, they would take a skin the size of a blanket and wrap the medicine man in it, squeezing him tightly from head to toe, like a cigar in a band.

Enclosed in this envelope was still wrapped around him, from the neck to the ankles, a large belt of raw skin, whose coils were no more than 2 or 3 cm apart, so that the wretch looked like a package.

It was not enough: at this point he was again wrapped in another skin and another belt tightened the body of the medicine man who was now completely immobilized.

Now, the medicine man lay helpless on the ground, looking like a long brown cigar.

He literally could not move a finger.

After that, the attendants would put him upright, trying to balance him on his bare feet.

He would stand there for a while as hard as a pole, then slowly begin to bend and rise on his knees and gradually each of these bends would turn into a jump that became longer and longer so that after a while the medical man would jump around the 4 poles with surprising speed, so much so that he looked like a phantom pole moving down in the air at such speed that his eyes could hardly follow it.

Then suddenly, with a great leap, so fast that no one could understand how the medical man could perform it, he landed heavily on the short clearing, maybe a foot wide, in the middle of the area occupied by the sharp pegs.

He had made a leap of about 3 meters flying over the dangerous pegs and landing safe and sound on the small clearing just enough to contain his feet. A great feat indeed.

But the really exciting part was yet to come.

As he stands there under the crossed poles, still tightly wound, our man sings the medicine song, accompanied by the roll of the big medicine drum, rhythmically played by his assistant.

What I am about to describe may seem strange: and strange it is, in fact, but that is exactly what happens.

How and why no one knows.

Almost immediately, as the medicine man stands there chanting his strange invocation to the spirits, voices are heard coming from above, voices that seem to descend from the opening made in the roof of the great medicine tepee,

Everyone can see that there is nothing up there but the night and the stars.

Where these voices come from, no Indian has ever been able to tell, but according to the medicine man, they are the voices of the spirits-the spirits with whom he is trying to communicate.

The most extraordinary thing here is that no one has ever been able to prove that it is anything else.

The voices express themselves in a language that we cannot understand, and not even the medical man can, except for a very few of them.

All he can say is that they speak in a foreign language, and that they are not the spirits he invokes.

There were only 4 spirits that our medicine man, White Dog, could understand.

I remember the name of only one: "First White Man".

And this name was invoked by our medicine men for years and years before our tribe learned that the white man really existed.

As the voices come wailing down into the hut, the medicine man rejects them one by one and continues to invoke one of the four spirits he can understand.

Sometimes it takes him a while to get it to come.

I even remember that a couple of times he failed to make contact and was forced to interrupt the ceremony, without having been able to achieve his goal.

But when he did make contact with the spirit he was looking for, he would fall into a state of excitement; we have seen some who would get up and start walking.

If what he wanted was information, the medicine man asked the question in an obscure form, known only to himself, and in an equally incomprehensible manner was given the answer, which he later had to translate for our use.

The answers were in our language, but expressed in such a way that we could not understand them and, as if that were not enough, it was the ancient way of speaking our language, as it was used many and many years ago, and only the oldest could grasp some phrases and some very old expressions.

But the scariest part of the ceremony for us kids took place at the end of the conversation between the medicine man and the spirits.

The conversations could end in many exciting ways, but the climactic scene was always accompanied by a raging wind, which would start howling through the roof of the hut as soon as the spirits had fallen silent.

Then the great medical tepee would shudder and sway under the lash of the wind that whistled through the rafters, making us tremble with fear.

It was an overwhelming finale.

A chaotic mixture of noises came down on us from above, from the round opening of the roof, whose beams stretched out into the night air. A pandemonium of voices that exceeded the moans of the wind, squeaks and rattles of who knows what objects and then suddenly, the whole hut shook, flames flickered, a terrifying scream of the medicine man was heard and then ...

Well, the medicine man disappeared before our eyes.

But soon after we heard him calling for help, and looking in the direction his voice came from, we saw him hanging by one foot from the roof of the hut, naked as a worm.

If he didn't fall and break his neck, it was only because of his foot, which, as far as we could see, was caught between the skin covering the tepee and one of the sloping beams that supported it.

"Kokenaytukhish pewow!" "Help! Screamed the medicine man like a madman.

And the spectators rushed in search of long poles, using which they removed him from that uncomfortable position, before he fell and broke his neck.

How he got up there no one knew; he claimed that it was the spirits who brought him up there as they left the tepee.

The Concept of Medicine for Native Americans

For Native Americans, the word "Medicine" meant much more than a substance to restore health and vitality to a sick or exhausted body.

Medicine meant "Power", the vital energy force contained in every aspect of nature, "completeness" and "wholeness". A person's Medicine was their energy, the expression of their vital organism. It also meant "Knowledge," because knowing gives a person the power to act.

"Medicine is anything that can help man feel more connected and in harmony with nature and all forms of life. Anything that heals the body, mind and spirit is Medicine. In order to find the answers to a particular problem, our Ancestors went into the forests to observe omens or signs that would assist them in the healing process. In this way they re-established a connection with the Allies (Higher Powers) and the Helpers of Medicine.

Medicine Man

Manitonquat is Medicine Man and spiritual leader of the Assonet Wampanoag. A great storyteller, he believes in the power that stories have to heal people, the community and therefore the Earth itself. He told me that very often people come to him asking him to teach them how to become shamans and if he says that it can take twenty or more years to teach what they want, they run away full of disappointment, looking for something faster. According to him, the people attracted to shamanism are just looking for something magical, along with the need to be recognized as someone who has power. They do not realize that they already have it. In any case, he adds, shaman is a word that comes from the ancient practices of the Native Siberians and only creates confusion by transferring terms from one culture to another.

Among the Lakota there are different types of Medicine men:

Wichasha wakan: literally: "sacred man". For an anthropologist it would be the classic "shaman". One can become one in many ways:

- he can be recognized as such from an early age, for particular habits that this child. In fact, he immediately appears different from his peers: he is more solitary, contemplative, "His eyes seem to look inside". His grandfather then begins to take him to ceremonies, tells him about the beliefs and traditions of his people and has a holy man instruct him in spiritual things.
- can receive power from an animal, either through a dream or as a result of a Vision Quest.
- may receive power from another wichasha wakan, at the time of his death.

Pejuta Wichasha: literally: "herb man." He is the classic medicine man who has the power to heal the sick. He must be able to speak the Lakota language, because language and religion are closely related. He must have the power to speak with the spirits and be able to speak the secret language of the shamans, the hambloglaka. He must know the right chants for each medicine he uses and those of the ceremonies he performs. If he does not know them or uses the wrong ones, everything he does will have no effect. He must have been instructed in his work by an older holy man. He must be sincere and know when he has power: power comes and goes, and can vanish in the twinkling of an eye. He can use one or several medicines; no one can know them all. He must have a few essentials for healing ceremonies: an eagle wing, a pipe bag, and a red stone pipe (for the Lakota). He must have a ceremonial rattle and drum to invoke the help of the spirits, and also sage, cedar, and sweet grass, which he will use for purifying fumigations. Each *pejuta wichasha* has his own Medicine Bag, with his medicinal herbs and sacred Medicine Objects.

He learns the secrets of the herbs from an expert or from dreams and visions. The Medicine of the Badger and the Bear are highly valued because they are considered four-legged *pejuta wichasha*.

A Medicine man knows where and from which direction to approach an herb, and whether it is effective during the day or at night. One should always harvest the whole plant, including the root, and never harvest a plant with seeds. An unceremoniously harvested plant will not heal anyone. It is able to place itself in the mind of the sick person and perceive their pain.

Among the Lakota, to ask for the help of a Medicine Man one must send him a red stone pipe, which he will then return. Some healings are performed spiritually through ceremonies, prayers, waving of eagle wings, and through the act of smoking the Sacred Pipe. No special medicine is administered in such cases. Other cures are performed by preparing a certain herbal tea, infusion or mush obtained from a special plant. Sometimes this procedure is combined with a Purification ceremony in the Sweat Lodge.

Yuwipi: "the discoverer", "the dreamer of the Rock", "the man of the flickering lights", "the one who is bound", "the man of the tracing stones": these are some Lakota expressions that designate this very mysterious figure, because of the special healing ceremony that only he can perform. We turn to him when a child has wandered off and is never found again, when something is lost or stolen, when a sick person wants to know the cause of his illness. Then the Yuwipi man arranges the Night Mystery, during which he, through his own personal Sacred Stone, will contact the spirits to know what he wishes to know. His stone is always perfectly round and often painted red, and is a "tracing stone". In this stone is embodied Tunka, the Rock, the Supernatural Power of the immovable. The Yuwipi man also uses gourd rattles, filled with 405 (number representing all the different types of plants present in the Lakota world) small crystals taken from the anthills: these are the "speaking stones", and their sound is the voice of the spirits.

Wapiya: he is a sorcerer and magician, feared and admired at the same time, depending on the use he makes of his power. With his positive nature he heals the sick, while in his negative aspect he is the "keeper of the bones", the evil sorcerer who causes diseases. A good Wapiya can use a wooden stick to pierce a vein and draw out the bad blood along with the disease, or he can suck it with his mouth directly from the body of the sick person and then spit it out.

Waayatan: is the prophet, the one who is able to see into the future and predict what will happen.

Heyoka: is the "opposite", the one who does everything backwards. Heyoka is the inversion of the expression hoka hey that the Native warriors shouted while launching themselves into battles. He is a "dreamer of Thunder", i.e. he must have dreamed of Wakinyan, the Birds of Thunder: dreaming of them automatically makes a man a heyoka, whether he wants to be or not.

His figure makes the fun in the sacred, but being a heyoka is not something to joke about because his power is immense: he can perform extraordinary *healings and even change the weather, when necessary (for example during very important rituals such as the Dance of the Sun).*

In the Seneca tradition it is never revealed which, among the members of the Nation, are the Persons of Medicine. A true Medicine Person never says, "I am a Medicine Man or Medicine Woman." Others may say it about someone else, but it is forbidden to declare it about oneself.

Lame Deer relates that his father used to tell him, "A wichasha wakan must be taller than an eagle and lower than a worm. He must have his feet on the ground, be human and, at the same time, something more than human."

At the Seneca a Medicine Person must have five requirements:

1. *he must be a Consultant, that is, assist others by helping them discover their own personal talents, their own Medicine and a good path to take in life. He must be able to impart Traditional solutions using Tribal Law and wisdom.*

2. *Must be a Historian of Earth Memories, i.e. know the stories of Creation and the first Four Worlds, as well as the prophecies of the future Fifth, Sixth and Seventh Worlds.*

3. *Must be an Herbalist/Healer, i.e. know the use of medicinal plants and natural healing cures derived from Mother Earth. The Herbalist also knows the Medicine of Creatures (animals) and how they assist Bipeds*

(humans) in finding spiritual or mental cures. This talent also includes the ability to recognize and diagnose diseases of body, mind and spirit.

4. *Must not have the personal Gift of Prophecy, i.e. must be a Seer, a Dreamer or otherwise be able to communicate with the Spirit World at will, since at any time the need may arise.*

5. *He must not have the ability to teach others all aspects of wisdom and knowledge. His experience must be shared so that Medicine can continue to live on and assist future generations.*

Fools Crow, who died in 1989, Ceremonial Chief of the Teton Sioux, considered by many to be the greatest Native American sacred man of the last hundred years, called Medicine People "hollow bones" through which Higher Powers operate. He told his biographer and friend Thomas E. Mails:

"The cleanest bones serve Wakan Tanka and the Higher Powers best; sacred people and medicine people work hard to become clean. The cleaner the bone, the more water can be poured into it and the faster it will flow.

Power comes to us first because we make ourselves what we are supposed to be, and then it flows through us to the outside world, to others. Power takes over in the life of a sacred person. It affects everything about us. We are able to heal ourselves and others. We can make journeys with our spirit to the abodes of the Higher Powers, and we can transform ourselves into animal creatures or birds that go among the people to see what is happening. But all Medicine People are different from ordinary people. The way they think is different. What happens to them is different. They understand things within themselves that others do not. It is these thoughts and this understanding that cause them to reach the heights of power necessary for their work. Our lives are a dance of power; our people see it and therefore honour us. I have never touched alcohol or drugs; I have not even used peyote as is the case in the Native American Church. Wakan Tanka is able to take me higher than any drug can."

Symbology of the Wheel

"The Medicine Wheel could be called a Circle of Knowledge that reconstitutes the Whole and empowers an individual's life."

It is sometimes called the Sacred Circle. From this simple definition it is possible to understand the two fundamental aspects of the Wheel: being both a mirror of the Universe and of man.

Through the symbolism of the Wheel it is possible to come into contact with and understand oneself and the world, according to the fundamental principle of the natives: "As it is inside, so it is outside".

It acts as a mirror: looking at it, one can see a reflection of the universe and of the Great Mystery, the Universal Mind that created everything that exists. One can read in it the functioning of the universe, coming to an understanding of the experiences of life and of the cosmic and natural laws, of the principles and forces that shape and animate human life.

In the Sacred Circle it is possible to see the interdependence of all things, thus discovering to be in relationship with everything, and thus deepening one's understanding of the Whole and of oneself.

The Wheel is a physical, mental, spiritual and emotional tool that allows those who use it to become attuned to the earth forces and natural energies that exert an action on their lives. The Native American sees the universe as a "becoming", that is a "coming-to-world", whose essence is not material but mental and spiritual. Everything that has manifested or is manifesting, has a purpose; and everything that exists (mineral, plant, animal or human) is made up of intelligent energy, held together by harmonious synchronization; everything is connected by vibrations of light, color, sound. Therefore, when a medical man builds a Circle containing any representation of physical objects, forces and energy, he actually builds a symbolic functional model of the way the Universal Mind, and therefore the human mind, operates. The one and the other are not only similar, but integrated.

Totems serve as connectors between different levels of consciousness: human, animal, vegetable, mineral. There is a network that allows the exchange of information between all life forms. Totems play the role of symbolic sensors by tapping into that network. Thus, we have animal, plant and mineral totems. Says Kenneth Meadows

" The plant kingdom feeds on trace elements that come from the mineral kingdom; by assimilating them, it allows inert minerals to evolve to a higher form of life and expression. Similarly, the plant kingdom serves as food for the animal kingdom, and thus continues its development. The fourth kingdom, the human kingdom, depends on minerals, plants and animals for its survival. The kingdoms are therefore states of existence, and when we connect to a totem, we connect with another state of existence that can help modify our own."

Each realm is connected to a particular direction in the Wheel.

Four Cardinal Directions

SOUTH

ELEMENT: WATER.

Physical water is fluid and if it is poured into a container it takes its shape: therefore it represents fluidity and adaptability.

Elemental Water also represents life: without the fluid and penetrating movement of water, the Earth would dry out and become arid and nothing could grow.

Similarly, humans without water would quickly die.

Our emotions and feelings are an expression of Elemental Water, which in native anatomy is linked to the belly, and like the Earth, man would become dry and fragile without the flow of emotions.

The celestial body associated with the South is the Moon, which is closely related to water: just think of the tides and menstrual cycles of women. But the Moon also influences the flow of sap in trees and plants, the fluids of the human body, blood pressure, brain fluids and pregnancy.

The South is related to Summer and the color Red, the color of oxygenated blood. It is associated with vitality, health, vigor, courage, physical energy and sexual power.

Human body: to the South are associated: blood, heart, blood circulation. In the Southeast the lymphatic system and endocrine glands. To the South-West the skin and muscles. To the South is related the sense of taste and therefore the mouth.

KINGDOM: VEGETABLE

The South is the realm of Giving, and plants are great givers of energy.

Plants and trees give themselves to the planet and offer themselves as nourishment and shelter to the creatures of the Animal and Human Kingdoms.

Plants and trees are living beings, and with their life force and mineral composition they help the healing processes. Each tree or plant has its own gifts, talents and abilities to share. Generally, a parallelism can always be drawn between the physical and emotional effects of the plant in question on man.

QUALITIES: TRUST AND INNOCENCE

The South is called "The Way of the Child." We are conceived in the South-East and born in the South, according to the vision of the Native man; then we grow up following the Wheel in a clockwise direction, touching the different directions according to the phases of our life. So the South corresponds to childhood, the West to adulthood, the wise North to old age and in the East there is the Golden Door that our spirit crosses at our death.

The Power of the South is the power of growth that follows birth.

The main characteristics of the child are trust and innocence, wonder and enthusiasm that make us see life as a wonderful experience.

On an emotional, mental and spiritual level, these are the healing avenues that this Direction can offer according to I Seneca:

- the spirit of play, the ability to laugh at what upsets one's pride, innocence and humility.

- the potential of the body, the development of its dexterity, listening to the body that allows it to express itself freely and not to develop tensions.

- confidence in one's own beauty and truth: " When you can destroy the illusion of who you are to others and truly be yourself you will have restored your innocence."

The South helps to reconnect with one's original essence and reclaim the "Dream to walk awake" that constitutes the purpose of our existence.

The South is the place of the unconscious and therefore associated with it are the fears related to childhood, those that may have remained crystallized within us, giving rise to the patterns Manitonquat speaks of. They are mental patterns that we have built to protect us when, as children, we have experienced dangerous situations or we have been injured. Created to react to a contingent suffering, they are then crystallized within us, in the unconscious, with the result that we use them indiscriminately. Our behavior can no longer be natural until we recognize the old wound and take care of it, understanding that whenever we do not act with love towards others, we are not in touch with our essence, which is made of love. By using our old pattern we are only showing how much we have been wounded. The South helps in this cleansing process, which is exactly what the aforementioned Fools Crow refers to when talking about empty bones.

The South is associated with man's emotions and their job is to give: if you give with your body or mind you create disharmony in our inner constitution. It is only by giving himself with emotions and feelings that man realizes his integrity. Love is the gift of self; the emotion that expresses the e-movement is love energy in motion. By blocking our emotions, man blocks his heart.

TOTEM: TOPO

The mouse represents the ability to become aware of things by approaching them with sensations and touch. The South teaches us to act in the same way, with confidence in our intuition, our sensations and our emotions, listening to them without repressing them, which would create a block and therefore an imbalance in the distribution of forces between the Four Directions.

WEST

ELEMENT: EARTH

The characteristics of the Elemental Earth are solidity, inertia, stability.

The West is the place of matter, appearances, the world of form, physical manifestation and the place of experience where we learn and grow. The Earth is often represented by its most enduring form, stone. The nature of the Earth is sustaining, giving comfort, constancy and security.

West is associated with Autumn and as a celestial body is linked to the Earth, while the color of the West is Black, the color of non-form from which everything originates. It absorbs all the colors of the spectrum in itself, stores and is protective. It is the receptive polarity of the solar spectrum and therefore it is a color related to the feminine aspect of human nature, to the intuitive sensitivity. Black were in fact the Tents of the Moon, the tepees where the Native women withdrew during menstruation, to listen in the depths of their body to the powerful contact with Mother Earth, which manifests itself with great strength through the woman's body during the cycle.

Human body: To the West are associated bones, skeleton, joints. It is linked to the sense of touch and therefore to the whole body.

KINGDOM: MINERAL

The Mineral Kingdom is considered the holder and controller of energy and is the oldest of the Kingdoms, as rocks and stones were on Earth before plants and animals. The Stone People hold the memories of Mother Earth. The function of the West is therefore to hold, to preserve, and is associated with the body. Through the body we are allowed to store energy and nourishment, but in the body we can also keep the old wounds that made us suffer in the emotions, mind or spirit and that are fixed here reaching a finally visible form: the disease.

For Medicine Men there is a link between the sensory organs of man and certain stones, which have the power to heal that particular organ to which they are connected. Crystals and stones also exert an action on the mental and emotional states of man and are very often used as healing tools.

QUALITIES: INTROSPECTION AND TRANSFORMATION

The West is the place of "looking within", of introspection heralding change. It indicates the power that comes from self-knowledge. It is the place of Death: it is nothing but a change, the passage to a new beginning.

The West is also the place of Dreams and Visions of the future. The Thunder Beings live here.

The color black associated with the West represents the Void that houses all answers.

The introspective capacity is the feminine energy, which is receptive.

Three are the paths of healing that the West offers us:

- introspection: this involves entering the stillness of our inner Sacred Space and listening to the teachings that come from our daily experiences. Here it is the receptive-feminine side that must be activated.

- Recognize one's own personal truth: This is the time to digest the answers that present themselves and learn to apply them.

- Walk your truth: Natives use the expression: "Walk your talk". With the knowledge that comes from experience, we can formulate a plan on how to achieve our goals. And if these are based on our personal truth and desire, then they can be approached with joy.

TOTEM: BEAR

The Grizzly, Grey Bear, is known for its great strength. The strength that this Totem allows us to contact is that of those who know how to recognize the right moment to withdraw to recover strength and reorganize their thoughts. Only in this way is it possible to prepare new and fertile strategies of action. Because of the great knowledge that the bear has of therapeutic herbs and of how to heal wounds, a medicine-man who dreams of the Bear becomes a bearer of Bear Medicine, which is precisely that of those who use herbs and plants to heal.

NORTH

ELEMENT: AIR

The characteristic of the Elemental Air is movement, constant change, often sudden, sometimes unexpected. It is lightness, freshness, freedom. Air carries "the breath of life" and is transformative. It carries our thoughts, dreams and aspirations. Therefore, Air is associated with the mind and with communication. It is also related to the wind that touches the soul of all living things and carries in its travels a particle of everything it touches. This element is associated to mental activity and communication.

The color of the North is white, the color of purity and balance. It is the sum of all colors of the solar spectrum and therefore represents perfection and completeness.

The North is then associated with winter and the stars, which for the Natives were a symbol of universality and divine protection. They believe they are descended from the Star People, who brought them to Earth millions of years ago.

Human body: To the North is associated the autonomic nervous system and breathing. To the North-East brain, nervous system and spine. To the Northwest is the peripheral nervous system. The North is related to the sense of smell and therefore to the nose.

KING: ANIMAL

The Natives believed that the animal also possessed a spirit and their more instinctive behavior allowed them a deep contact with the environment. Observing animals, the Natives learned many things about trees and plants, about their food and medicinal uses, but they also recognized that each animal was the bearer of a special teaching. Through animal totems it is possible for man to contact the power, the Medicine of each animal, listening to what it can communicate to the human soul.

Animals are considered "receptors" of energy and can therefore transmit it to the human mind. The function of the North is in fact to receive: it is the human mind that has the function to receive information from outside. If we use the body, we can only receive material things, using emotions we risk to be continuously hurt, while with the mind we are in contact with the Universal Mind and with the meanings that it has distributed in everything that exists. Our mind also provides the protections that we need in our relationships with the world.

QUALITIES: KNOWLEDGE AND WISDOM

The North is the Place of the Elders, of knowledge and wisdom. Knowledge means "what is known" and for the Natives it includes philosophy, religion, science, which must be integrated with each other in life.

With this Direction is also associated the gratitude for the continuous understandings that occur in the process of growth and for the 16 Supernatural Powers that support us continuously. Thankfulness and gratitude towards all that exists is very important, according to the Natives, to maintain harmony with all our Relations.

TOTEM: BISON

The Bison was the most important animal for Native Americans because it gave itself completely to allow man to live, providing him with everything he needed.

It symbolized the Spirit that gives all of itself and its essence for the process of life.

It was also the symbol of man's dependence on Nature for his survival and therefore the necessary gratitude for that.

EAST

ELEMENT: FIRE

Fire is the radiant energy of the Universe, the spark of life. On a human level it is expressed by enthusiasm, the drive to improve and resourcefulness. Fire is a very powerful element: it has the characteristics of expansion, rapidity, destruction that precedes regeneration. It is what gives energy to our physical body, through digestive combustion.

According to ancient wisdom, the entire Universe is Fire in the process of transformation. Everything in the Universe was considered condensed Fire, solidified light. The color of the East is therefore Yellow, the season is Spring, and the celestial body associated with it is the Sun. These three things are symbols of life, of continuous transformation and regeneration, of Illumination and inner light.

Fire was associated with the spirit, and in fact Nature was seen as the condensation, the material manifestation of the Great Spirit.

Human Body: To the East is linked the reproductive system.

KINGDOM: HUMAN

The East is linked to Man, the only living being to whom the Great Mystery has given Self-awareness. Every man, in life, chooses to use, with intention, his strengths in a positive or negative, constructive or destructive way. Motivation is everything. The main function of the East is precisely to determine, choose and decide how to use the energies that are available to each. To maintain the balance between the Directions, man should make his decisions with the spirit, which is directed by the intelligence, which in turn is transmitted by the mind. Thus the spirit has a mental power and consciousness. The human soul is the abode of the individualized spirit; it is the system of manifestation of life that makes it possible for the spirit, individual essence and inner identity, to express itself on all levels. It is the soul that holds the experiences of life, and these can lead man to accumulate power within himself.

QUALITY: ENLIGHTENMENT

The East was called by the Natives "The Place of the Long View", because here one could have a "panoramic" view of life. Here is in fact the Golden Door that man crosses at his death.

The Power of the East is the Power of Light, of mental and spiritual enlightenment and of the inner vision that comes from the consciousness of the unity of all living things and that gives us courage.

The healing ways to which the East is related, according to the Seneca are:

- Creativity: by enhancing one's talents, one's essence is illuminated and given a voice.
- Healing and "transmutation of the poison", that is, using our innate power of self-healing to bring about the transformations necessary for our spirit to free itself and become more and more fully realized.
- The right use and exchange of one's own power: this is about understanding the right way to use one's own strength and energy. The real lesson of this path is that the true energy exchange is sharing.

East retains the energy of the masculine side of human nature, the side that chooses and acts with independence and clarity.

TOTEM: EAGLE

The Eagle is the symbol of freedom from all forms of ignorance and bigotry, of clairvoyance and prescience. It guards the home of the noblest ideals, it is closest to Grandfather Sun and bathes in the love of his light; the Eagle is able to look directly at the Sun without being dazzled by it.

The Eagle also teaches balance, because even the loss of a single feather from one wing is compensated for by the loss of a feather from the other wing as well.

The Eagle symbolizes the importance of principles, that is, the fundamental truths, the essential spirit, the profound intention that guides action.

While each medicine man develops his own personal way of using the Wheel of Four Directions, there are some procedures common to all. One can use for concentration the typical willow circle, with a diameter of about 35 *centimetres, with directional laces, colored cloth flaps, some totemic objects such as bird feathers, bear nails, eagle claws, as symbolic sensors able to connect with the Medicine of that particular animal. Purifying fumigations are always made with sage, cedar or sweet grass and often people smoke the Pipa, a ritual instrument that creates a deep contact with the Helpers, through the smoke - connected to the Air element and therefore to the Universal Mind, to the wisdom and knowledge of the North. It is necessary to purify one's mind from superfluous thoughts, creating an empty and calm mental space, relaxing completely and closing the eyes. The intention to call the help of the Four Directions regarding a particular problem must be very clear and precise. At this point, in a condition of openness and receptivity, presence and attention, the thought dwells on each Direction, connecting with the Entity that lives there, the Helper. You use its power to form thoughts, sensations and images that bring clarification to your problem. It tells you not only where the problem is and what is the cause, but also what other Entities to call for treatment and what to give more importance to. In the case of an illness it is very important to determine its cause, otherwise the evil may return. Many medicine men use crystals to achieve clarity and very deep connections with the Entity.*

Fools Crow before embarking on a process of caring for a person, he would make deep contact with them to see how great their faith in caring was. He also posited the difference between curing and healing: "Curing is something spiritual, but not as much as healing. People die. Not everyone gets cured. I have not asked Wakan Tanka why this is so. I also know that He does not remove a person from this world. That would make Him responsible for all deaths, including the tragic ones. If it seems to Him that they cannot, or should not be cured, for whatever reason, He may decide not to interfere or change the situation. He just lets them come to Him. There are occasions, however, when He decides to interfere and keep the patient alive." In the event that the person could be healed, Fools Crow would talk with them at length to understand their life and anything that was important to the healing. It was very important to convey to the patient a deep sense of peace, of trust, of freedom from fear, all of which profoundly affect the very possibility of the cure and its strength. In order to get in touch with the Directions, the simplest thing he did was to make a small altar on the ground, marking the four corners with pieces of cloth in the colors of the Directions, placing between them a bed of sage on which he sat, wrapped in a black blanket, so that in his mind a black screen would form through which he could receive the information he needed. Then he prayed, asking for help from the Entities and Wakan Tanka, holding his own Medicine Stone in his hand. In a short time he got an understanding of the problem, what had caused it, which medicine to use, how to prepare and apply it, which ceremonies to perform, in case herbs and ointments were not enough. Smells and sounds were always part of the cure: "The nose stimulates memory and connects us to the past. Smells are associated with everything we do. Wakan Tanka covered the Earth with smells. Sweet ones, such as sweetgrass or sage, are protective in the sense that they ward off evil. Smells also cause us to experience feelings, emotions, desires, and inspirations. In addition, everything that exists has a sound. Wakan Tanka, Grandmother Earth and the other Helpers use sounds to communicate with us, sometimes with words, but more often to stimulate our minds and hearts to think about spiritual things. Grandmother Earth speaks to us through the drum. The rattles are the gentle voice of Wakan Tanka sending cascades of blessings upon the earth. The flutes are the many voices of the Entities of the Directions. Thunder is the powerful voice of the Beings of the Clouds. It is to the ears that the stones speak first and through the ears of the mind, spirit and heart." Fools Crow implemented the healing practices four times a day for four days, using herbs in the form of infusions, ointments made with animal fat and pigments of the colors of the Four Directions to be applied directly on the body, chants, musical instruments, traditional ceremonies such as the sweat lodge, depending on the type of problem that the patient presented and the instructions given by the Helpers. Each medicine man has his own personal means of healing, developed during his own Path of Knowledge. For Fools Crow it was very important to communicate to the person his deep love: "The person has to feel it, has to know that everything I'm doing is sent to him in the form of baskets full of love. Then, when love has reached her, her own love for me will begin to grow and when the care is over we are closer than if we were brother and sister. Our love is unity of mind, heart and spirit." For Fools Crow, a very important step of healing is also to release anger and grief so as to create within oneself the space necessary to listen to Wakan Tanka and the Helpers. He strongly believes in the ability of self-healing that every man has: according to him the body is something extraordinary and most diseases could be cured by itself, without the intervention of a person-medicine. He believes that the way a person thinks can make the body sick or keep it in shape, although this does not include all types of diseases, such as contagious ones, severe burns and wounds. Balance is also important with regard to disease, he even says it is the best antidote to disease. If we maintain harmony between the Four Directions within us, the body, the mind, the emotions and the spirit, there can only be harmony in our relationships with the outside of us: other people, the Earth, the Great Mystery. This is health according to the Natives: honoring the Sacred Circle that unites everyone with everything that exists.

Fools Crow knew, however, that the effectiveness of a cure was the result of the combination of the work of the Higher Powers, the person-medicine, the medicine itself, and the procedure followed. Spiritual power was its central levitating ingredient. Fire, sage, sweet grass and music made their contribution. The support of family and friends was also essential: their attitude should focus on encouraging the patient to focus on his own life and life in general. Even the environment in which the treatment was performed played its role. The better it was, the more profound and rapid the results would be. Fools Crow rejected the idea that the medicines used by the Sioux had come to them through a series of trials and errors. For him, this was tantamount to saying that the best thing Wakan Tanka could do for the men was to leave them to their own devices, or that perhaps there was no power. Admitting the experimental method would have implicitly meant that Wakan Tanka didn't care enough about the people He had created to provide them with guidance over the centuries, and that He was leaving them to suffer and die until the experimental process was complete. Said Fools Crow: "To accept such a thing would make the Higher Powers look like monsters instead of loving Beings. I and all the other medicine people have been and are guided by Wakan Tanka and the Helpers to the plants we need for treatment. Just as they are involved in all methods of treatment, so they are part of the process of choosing plants. What I take out of my Medicine bundle or get from the fields and forests is not something accidental. I use a lot of medicine, but I have never given someone medicine that made them sicker or caused any side effects. Only white people's medicine does that. They prescribe us something as if the same medicine works for everyone in the same way. Only when the person gets worse do they try to give you a different kind of pill or something else. Many times they mix different pills or medications and they have absolutely no idea what will happen. This never happens among us, but most of our people have been persuaded for a long time to stop coming to us for treatment. One day, however, everyone will realize that the best way to cure is to combine the essence of what we do with what white doctors do. Then the cure will be truly great."

Yana Nashua

BOOK 2

Native American Apothecary

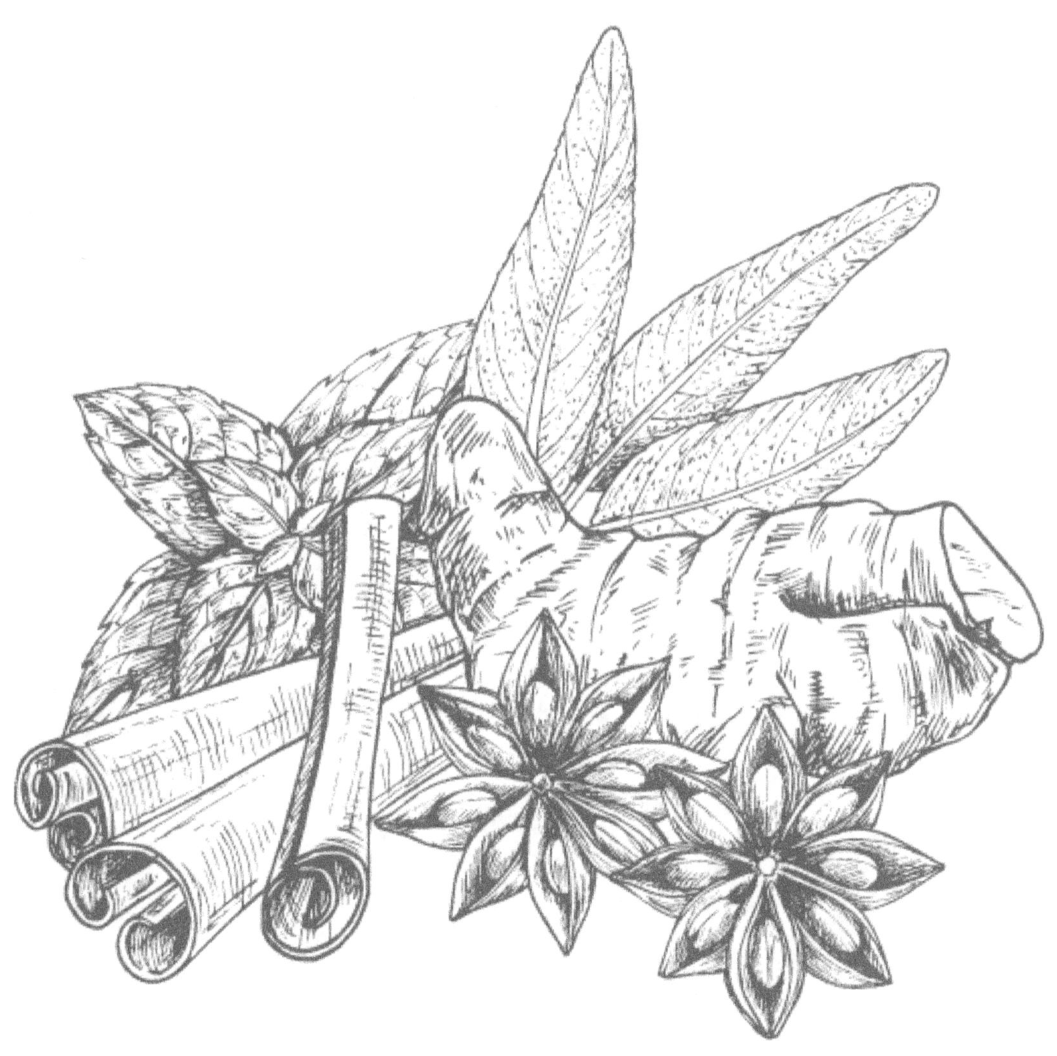

Native Americans and the Use of Stimulant Plants and Hallucinogens

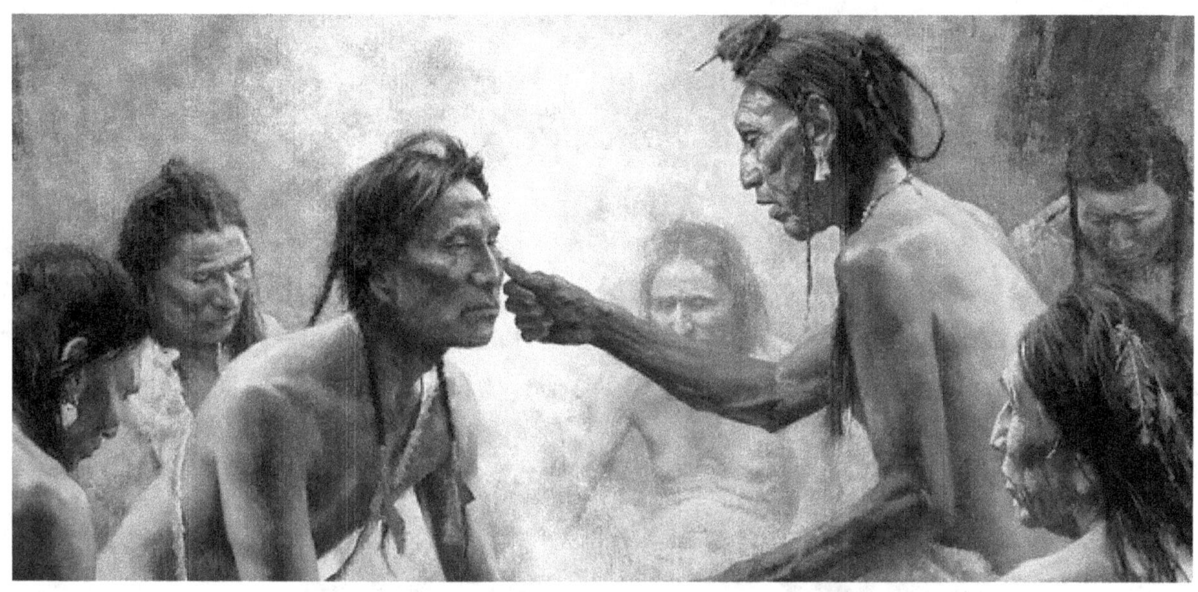

It is known to all the scholars of Native American cultures that American Indians used a great variety of plants, among which some wild and some cultivated, both for religious and practical purposes and for simple pleasure or taste. As for religion and the many rituals that characterized the community life of natives, the hallucinogenic qualities of certain substances certainly facilitated the search of visions and the "contact" with the world of spirits. Other applications were purely medical, as psychotropic plants - as they are scientifically called - were used as remedies and painkillers or stimulants, in cases where the same substances were used to increase energy and courage; finally, they also had a social function because the use of substances in common, created bonds of friendship and loyalty.

In many cases, especially in periods of war and pacification, they served both ritualistic and practical purposes, and certain pleasant sensations derived from certain applications.

South American Indians made use of different psychotropic plants, of which the most known was the coca leaf from which cocaine was derived. In North and Central America the major stimulants, intoxicants and hallucinogens were tobacco, alcoholic beverages, peyote, stramonium, mushrooms, mescal, black drink and ololiuqui.

Tobacco

Already some generations after the arrival of Columbus, the use and cultivation of tobacco known in Europe through the Arawaks, West Indian Indians, spread in many regions of the world.

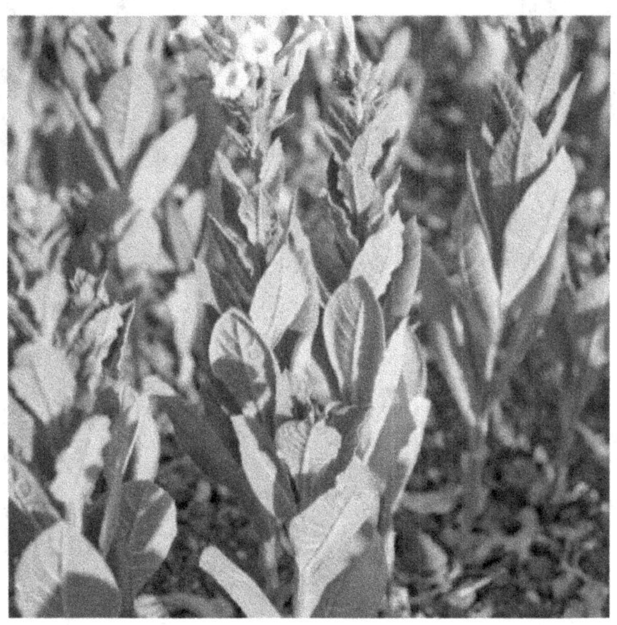

The word tobacco is the Spanish version of the Arawakan term for cigar. There are more than a dozen known types of this plant, but only a few are original to South America. Knowledge of the plant probably spread from south to north, along with agriculture and corn. Based on the archaeological sites, we can assume the beginning of tobacco use as early as before "Contact".

Tobacco and the Pipe

Later on an extensive cultivation of the plant was introduced and with it the use of the pipe. Besides being smoked (even mixed with other plants), tobacco was also chewed, sniffed and mixed with drinks. The Indians of all the regions of North America, except for the Arctic and some subarctic areas and the Columbia Plateau, used tobacco in one form or another, even before the arrival of whites who spread the use of the plant through their merchants in those regions as well.

Smoking, sniffing or eating tobacco was part of a ritual concerning war, peace, harvest, puberty and death. Indians burned the plant as incense, scattered its leaves or buried them with the dead. Many of these uses give the impression that they were sacrificial offerings. Religious applications included arousal in times of tension such as war or work, aesthetic purposes, physical comfort, and entertainment. The physiologically active alkaloid in tobacco is nicotine.

Alcoholic Beverages

For many North American Indians the consumption of alcohol was a phenomenon that arose after the "Contact", that is after the arrival of the white man. In fact, alcohol played an important role in the relationships between Indians and Europeans: it served as a commercial commodity in exchange for furs, to deceive Indians in negotiations, and as a catalyst for unrest and violence; however, in certain regions of the continent, after agriculture, the use of alcohol was highly developed, and in Mesoamerica, in the circum-Caribbean area and in the Southwest it was also used on a large scale already in times preceding the "Contact".

Indian alcoholic beverages were made from both cultivated and wild plants. There were at least 40 different kinds in Mexico alone...such as wheat beer, maguey and sotol wine, and berries, a drink made from fermented honey. Southwest Indians made drinks from cactus and Southeastern peoples from khaki. In many areas of the Southwest, among the Zuni, Yuman, and Apache, as well as in the Southeast, the use of alcohol was mostly unknown. However, the Papago and Pima of the Southwest believed that the consumption of alcoholic beverages brought rain. Among the Aztecs, intoxication served to induce meditation and prophecy. Public drunkenness was frowned upon and in some cases, even high class Indians were sentenced to death as commoners.

The Peyote

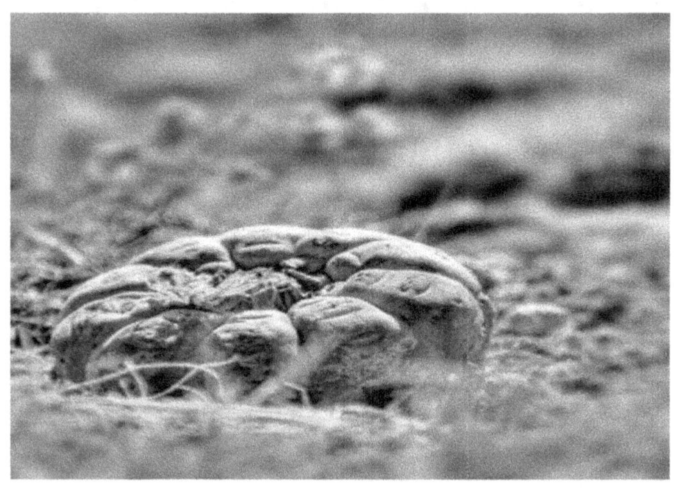

Peyote is the fruit of *Lophophora williamsii*, a small fleshy cactus without thorns which grows in the rocky deserts and among the mountains of northern Mexico, whose powerful hallucinogenic properties were known to the Aztecs who used it in many ceremonies, the botanical description dates back to 1845 classifying it as *Echinocactus Williamisii* and later *Anhoalonium Lewini*, belonging to the genus *Lophaphora* of *Cactaceae*. Dark blue-green, white or pinkish in color and globular in shape, it grows in the semi-desert regions of northern and central Mexico, and in the southern United States. Being a cactus, it grows without difficulty even in very hot environments and requires very little water and a minimal supply of nutrients. In the first phase of life peyote is covered with small spines which *are progressively replaced by woolly extensions. The flowers are generally similar to small daisies of a pale white or pinkish color.*

In its natural state peyote rarely emerges from the ground for more than 2-3 cm., the root of the plant is buried (up to a depth of 20 - 25 cm.). The part that comes out of the ground (commonly called 'boton') is the one that is cut and consumed either fresh or dried. The first news about its existence were given by Spanish chroniclers in the sixteenth century who talked about it as a plant having diabolic properties, then the royal doctor Francisco Hérnandez studied its properties and classified it as a medicinal plant calling it Peyotl Zacatencis, however the Viceroy of Spain tried to eradicate its religious use among the Aztecs and other natives by prohibiting it with scarce results and the ceremonies of peyote survived to every persecution. In fact prolonged and extremely violent attempts to eradicate its consumption failed, to the point that its use ended up spreading from the south of Mexico, across North America, to the central-western plains of the continent up to Canada. But no more than 150 years ago, peyote consumption in the United States could be punished by hanging. However, it too has been Christianized among converted Sierra natives and has become Peyotl's Santo Nino, but its ancient mythological origin remains as Juculi, the plant that Sun Father Ono Rugame left for men to cure their ills when he left the earth and is the only means of communicating directly with deities and spirits.

The response to the official efforts to eradicate the use of peyote was the creation of a formal church (the Native American Church, or NAC) that, after a very long legal dispute, was recognized by the legislative bodies the right to continue to celebrate the religious rites of the aboriginal peoples of pre-Columbian America, including ceremonies based on the collective use of peyote. Even today, NAC liturgical gatherings take place in tents in the desert after the sun goes down. Here peyote is consumed during the night and all participants ask the gods for the strength they need to be better Human Beings, to face the problems that afflict them (alcoholism, addiction, infirmity, disease) and to divine the future. It produces visions of various types: lights, colors up to true hallucinations that begin with a great well-being, extreme sensitivity and relaxation that promotes introspective awareness; after about three hours can begin the chromatic and geometric visions that are transformed up to fantastic images, depending on the availability and perception of the person who ingests it. For the Tarahumara it is a prodigious plant that possesses an Iwigla soul, it talks and sings while growing and it is recognized by the peyoteros. Some swear they have conversed with it during transport after harvesting, which is always preceded by abstinence and purification rites to enter the sacred areas where it grows and that only the great shamans know. During the harvesting, the shamans and the peyoteros assistants ingest small quantities of fresh peyote accompanied by large drinks of tesguino around a small cross and a fire performing the dutuburi and other sacred dances, then they return to the village to sell a part of the harvest celebrated by the whole community, but the plant acquires its full properties with the drying that precedes its consecration in a secret cave and from that moment can only be used by shamans. During preservation, peyote is offered food, beverages and tobacco, while it acquires its hallucinogenic and magical properties which could also cause death to those who touch it without being initiated.

When it is ready to be used for ceremonial or curative purposes, a cow is sacrificed and a feast is celebrated with libations and drinking of tesguino that precede the sacred dutuburi dances around three crosses in a sacred space and if the ceremony is important, the initiate sacred Matachines dancers also participate. Not far away two other crosses are planted dedicated to God and to peyote, in front of which the pot containing it is placed, then the ox sacrificed and destined to the peyoteros is brought to pieces, while the dance of peyote hikuli nawakebo is performed around the fire and that precedes the ingestion of the hallucinogen accompanied by the tesguino, after which everyone forms a circle in the center of which the shaman rhythms with his stick on the pot containing the plant and the dance begins again in pairs alternating the Duturbi with the Matachine until dawn. As soon as daylight the effect of peyote has worn off and, after everyone has eaten and drunk tesguino, the shaman begins the treatment of the patients by lightly hitting them on the head with his sacred stick and to each one he indicates the remedies for his disease, finally, he performs some magical movements with the staff facing the sun which rises three times and everyone washes their face and hands to purify themselves, then the light spreads over the mountains and penetrates the gorges and ravines, the Barranca del Cobre opens magnificently to the day along with the other canyons and the Sierra Madre wakes up while the spirits of the Tarahumara dissolve in their ethereal shelters. dissolve in their ethereal shelters. To this day, Mexican law ensures the right to possess and consume peyote for religious purposes only to members of the NAC, who have at least 25% Indian blood.

Stramonium

Stramonium or Datura is a tall, rough, annual growing plant belonging to the Solanaceae family. The Indians of Central America, the Southwest and California used the plant, usually as a tea, after grinding and soaking the leaves, stems and roots, in order to obtain an effect like the one obtainable with the consumption of peyote. In Mexico stramonium was sometimes used together with peyote, but elsewhere they each had their own culture. As in the case of peyote, its use was both secular and religious.

Medicinal use included use as an anesthetic for operations and as an ingredient in ointments.

The popular name, in America, of stramonium "jimsonweed" comes from "Jamestown weed", which English soldiers in Virginia in 1676 gave to the plant whose leaves they ate without knowing its consequences. However, there is no evidence that Southeastern Indians used stramonium for its psychoactive properties.

Other psychotropic plants

The term mescal is sometimes used for mescaline, an alkaloid of peyote, as well as for maguey (agave). However, the real mescal or "red bean", *Sophora secundiflora* belongs to the bean family (*Fabaceae*) and contains sulfurine, an alkaloid having an effect similar to that of nicotine. Various peoples of the Southwest, the Great Plains, and a small group in the Southeast ate mescal beans.

The use of the emetic "black drink" was uniquely a Southeastern phenomenon, with the exception of the Karankawa, Texas Indians, who are considered part of the Southwestern cultural area. The main ingredient in the drink was the plant *Ilex* (or *Ilex vomitoria*). Sometimes tobacco was also added. The Indians drank the "black drink" ritually as a purgative or stimulant of purification and inspiration before meetings, funerals, wars, or seasonal ceremonies such as the cue ritual (Busk ritual), also called the Green Corn Festival (Green Com Festival), an annual renewal ritual.

NATIVE AMERICAN MEDICINAL HERBS

Compass or pilot plant

The root of this plant can be found above the ground and is applied over the wounds caused If it is burned it causes a very thick smoke and can be inhaled for headache treatment purposes.

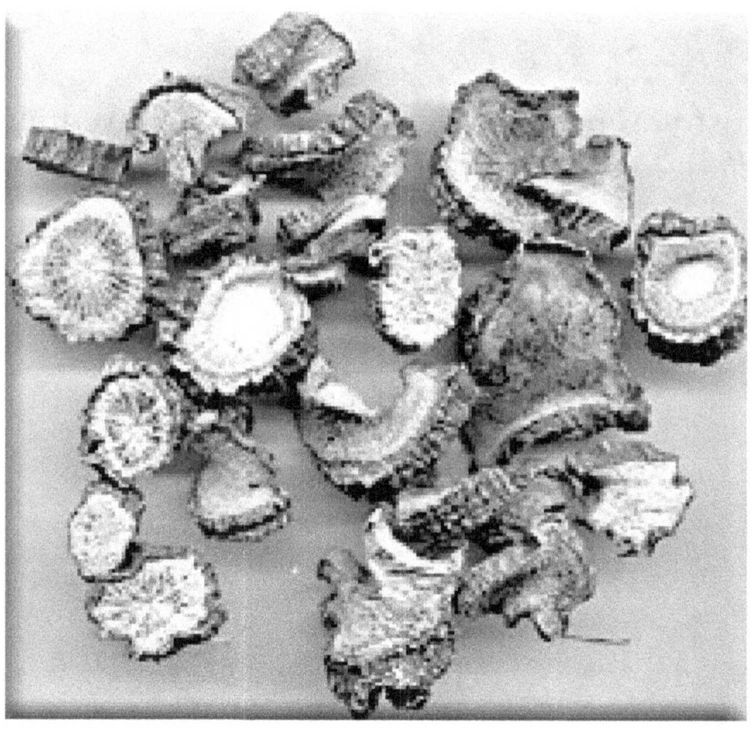

It is also used extensively over hot rocks in the sweat lodge.

Sweet flag root or bitterroot (sinkpe tawote; acorus calamus)

This root is one of the major medicines of the Lakota people. it is chewed to cure toothache and when prepared as an herbal tea it cures sore throats.

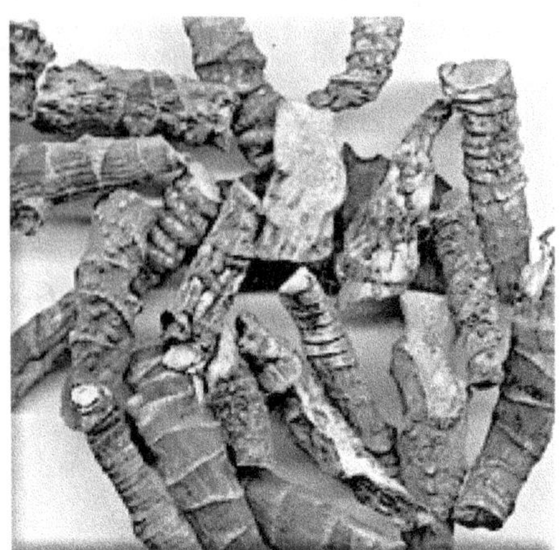

It is also chewed and placed on hot stones inside the sweat lodge so as to cause a decongestant steam: it is also chewed by singers to bring energy to their voices.

Bearberry leaf (wahpe canli; arcostaphylos uva ursi)

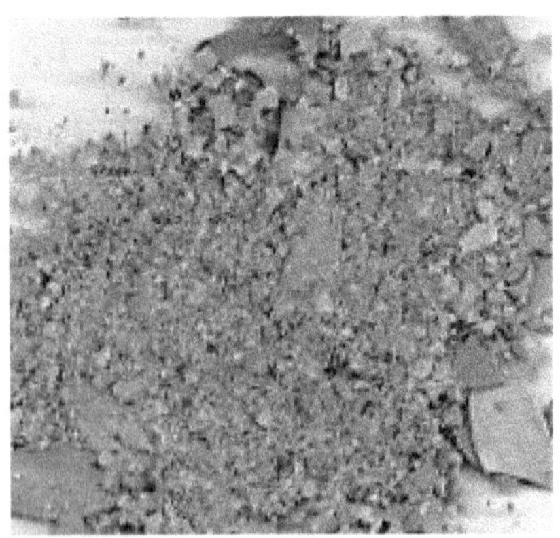

Also known as Kinnikinnick, these bagged and chopped leaves are mixed with cansasa and/or tobacco to make a mixture for smoking.

Bloodroot -sanguinaria canadensis

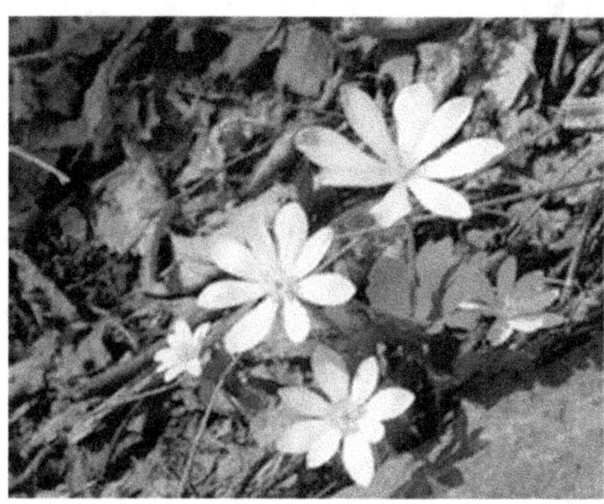

Bloodroot is a plant native to the eastern United States and parts of Canada. It is scientifically known as Sanguinaria canadensis. Bloodroot may also be called red root, raccoon root, terrorwort, Indian paint, and snakebite. It has a long history of use in both Native American medicine and modern chemistry and medicine.

Native Americans in the eastern United States used bloodroot to address lesions on the skin, such as tumours or warts. Bloodroot juice was also thought to purify the blood and was sometimes taken internally to soothe coughs. It may also have been used in higher doses to induce vomiting.

Flat cedar (hanble blaska; thuja occidentalis)

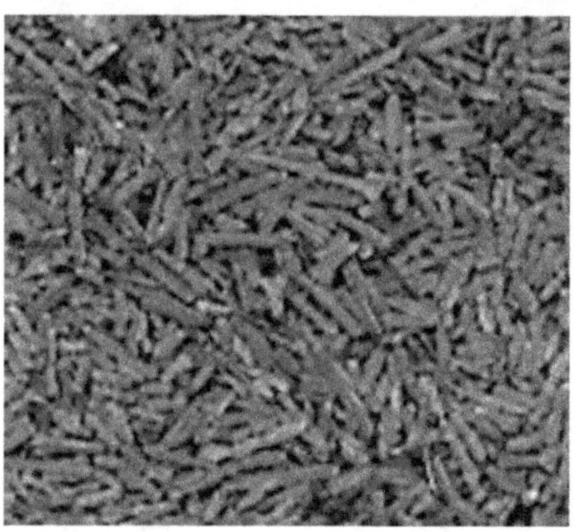

Although this plant is not found in the native area it is the preferred species of cedar to burn as incense for purification during ceremonies.

Lead plant (zitkata can; amorpha canescens)

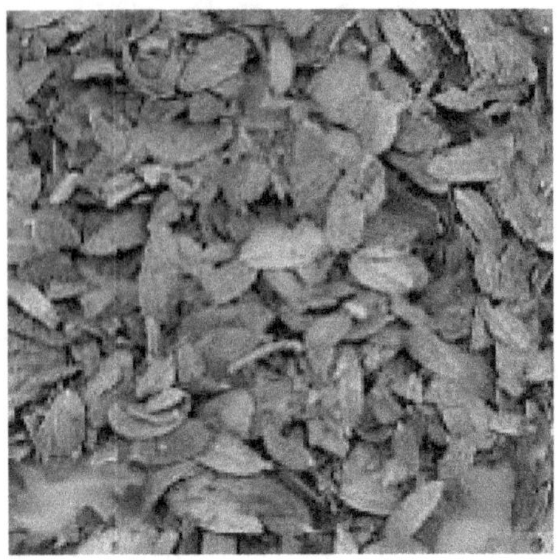

Tear and wet from the leaves to the central flower was used to relieve indigestion and coughs.

Lovage root (canli icahye)

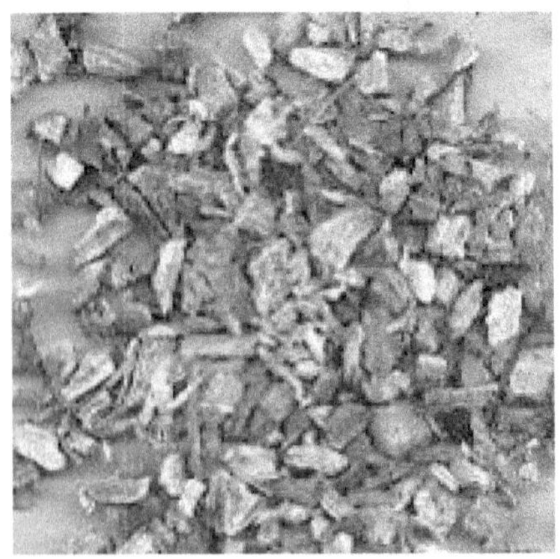

Also known as bear root, a small amount of this root mixed with cansasa, bearberry and/or tobacco make entirely a delicious flavor and a traditional blend to smoke.

Osha root

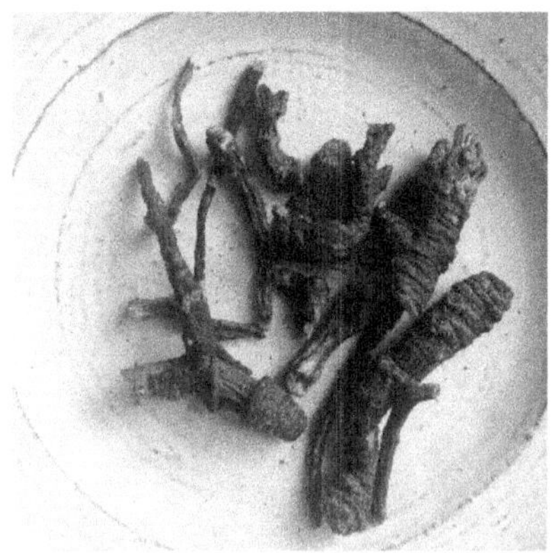

An aromatic root used to relieve coughs and sore throats, also known as snake root and spider root.

Sometimes used to flavor smoking mixes. Found at the top of the Rocky Mountains.

Red willow bark (cansasa; cornus amomomm, cornus stoloni fera)

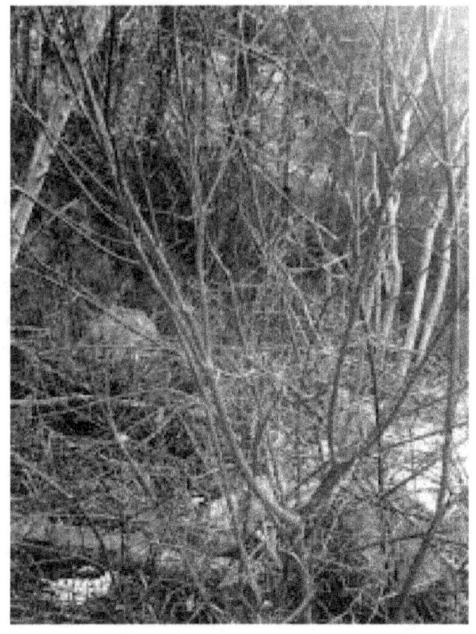

The bark of the red willow is scraped off the inside and the basic ingredient of the traditional smoking mixture is obtained. Cansasa is commonly mixed with bearberry and a small piece of lovage root.

Sage (peji hota; artemisia ludoviciana)

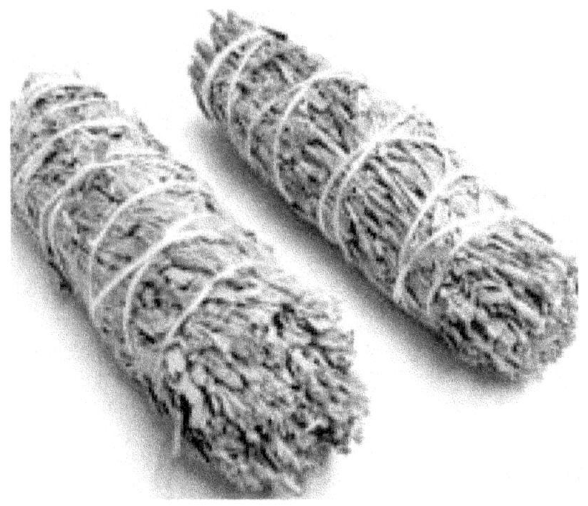

Sage is a plant that grows throughout the prairie. It is available seasonally. It is another medicine commonly used by all prairie tribes, it is burned to create a smoke used for purification. It is used in virtually every ceremony.

Sassafras bark (can hansa; laurus sassafras)

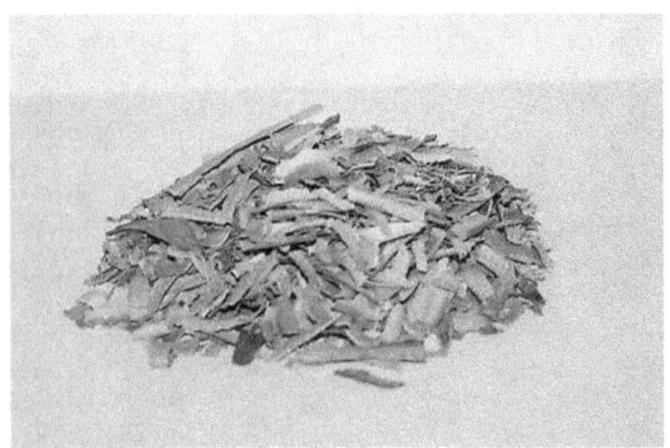

Eastern tribes used this aromatic bark to make an infusion to purify the blood and as a general tonic. Excellent taste.

Sumac (canzi; rhus glabra)

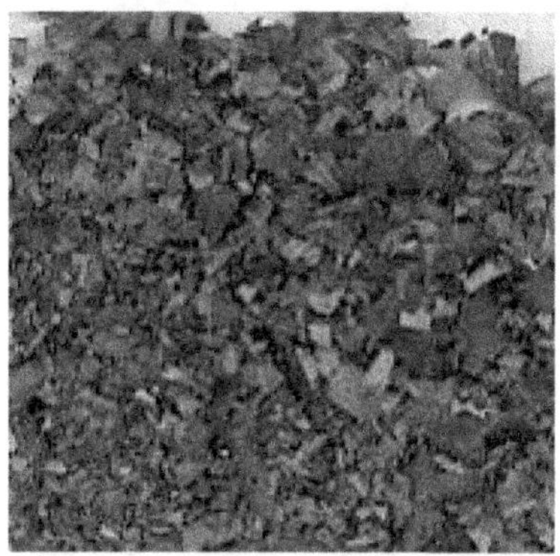

These leaves were used as a personal flavor in smoking mixtures.

Sweet grass (peji wakanga; hierochloe odorata)

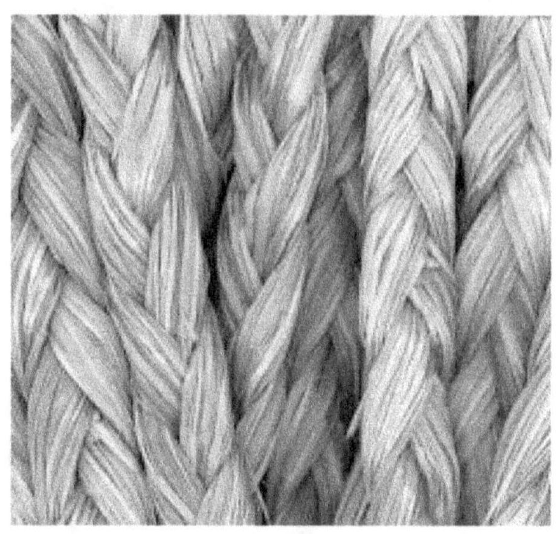

Burned it produces a sweet scent, used to purify along with sage in ceremonies is part of the traditional equipment placed in a medicine bag.

Gumweed (pte ici yuha; grindelia squarrosa)

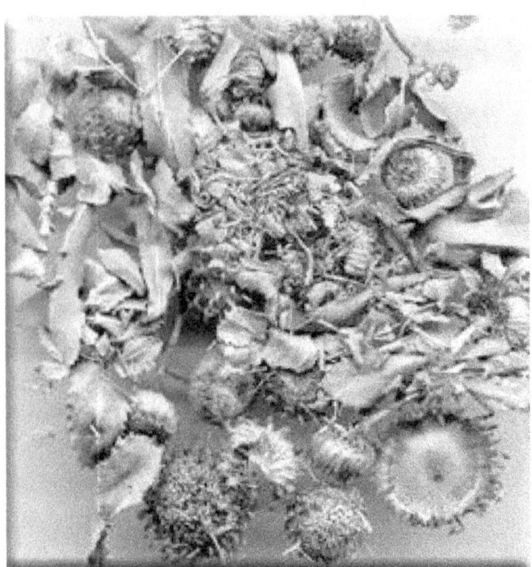

Herbal tea prepared with leaves and flower used to relieve indigestion and coughs.

Vervaine (pejuta to; verbena hastata)

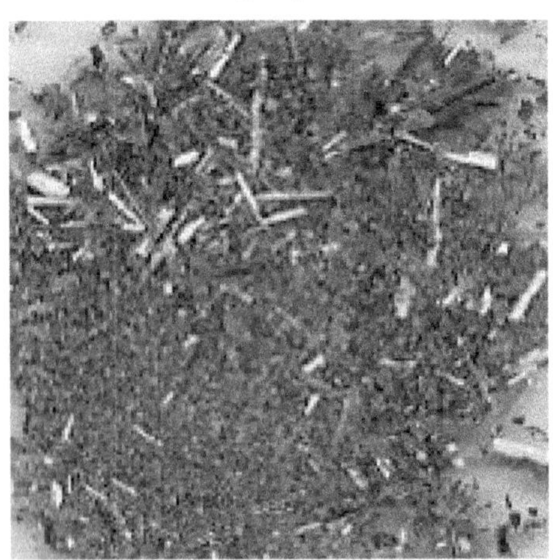

Infusion prepared with leaves and flowers used for drowsiness and to protect oneself from the cold.

Yana Nashua

The forgotten herbal cures of Native Americans

When it comes to herbal remedies, many of us are familiar with the benefits of Echinacea as an antibiotic, willow bark as a pain reliever, and aloe as a local anesthetic and treatment for skin conditions. But this is common knowledge compared to the insights and treatments that Native American medicine men discovered and used.

Native American medicine men developed a wheel much like the yin/yang of Asian medicine. The use of herbal remedies and other alternative forms of treatment was the cutting edge medicine of their day. This was a holistic approach to medical care that relied on plants and their unique benefits.

What follows is the list of native plants, trees, fruits and flowers unique to North America that have amazing benefits as defined by Native Americans.

These ancient cures are also good for everyday needs when you consider how effective some of them can be.

Licorice tea for a sore throat is a good example. It is also interesting that many of these natural cures are still in use today, including beeswax and bee pollen, chamomile and others. It is a good demonstration of the benefits of wisdom developed over the centuries.

It is difficult to know how the Native Americans determined that plants could have medicinal properties, although trial and error was probably one approach. It is also thought that they observed sick animals eating certain plants and determined that those plants must have some property worth exploring.

These drugs were generally administered via tea or pastes that were either ingested or applied externally. Sometimes the plants were consumed as food or added to food or water. Sometimes an ointment or poultice was applied to open wounds. Which I highly recommend you avoid these, given the risk of infection from wild sources.

Instead of endlessly listing plants that treat the same conditions over and over again, I have tried to isolate this grouping to the most common plants that can be found and recognized. As always, if you are pregnant, consult your doctor and do a lot of research before using any of these.

Alfalfa Herb

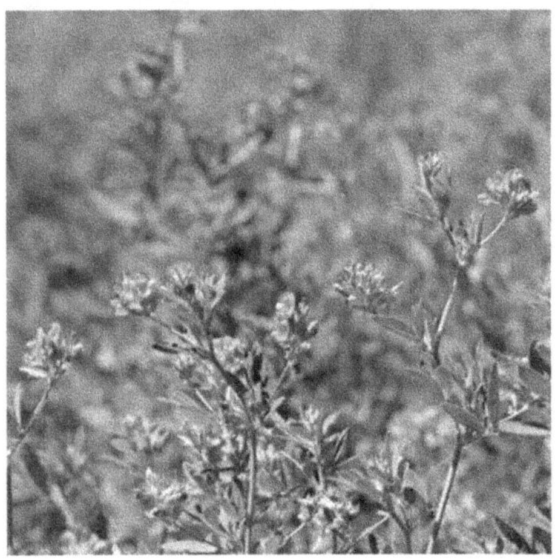

Relieves digestion and is used to help with blood clotting. Contemporary uses included treatment of arthritis, bladder and kidney conditions and bone strength. Strengthens the immune system.

Aloe

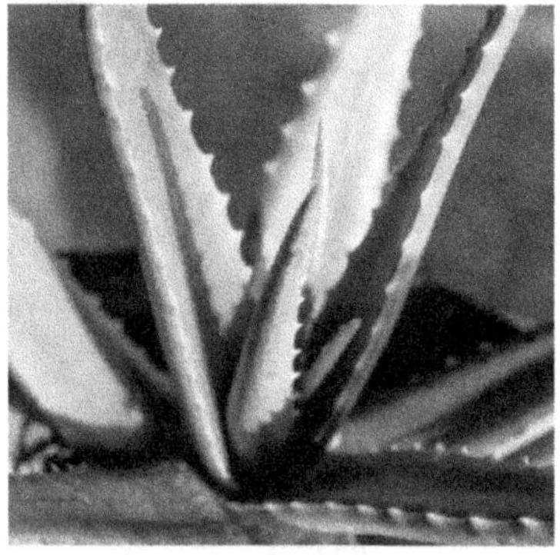

A cactus-like plant. The thick leaves can be squeezed to extrude a thick sap that can be used to treat burns, insect bites and wounds.

Aspen

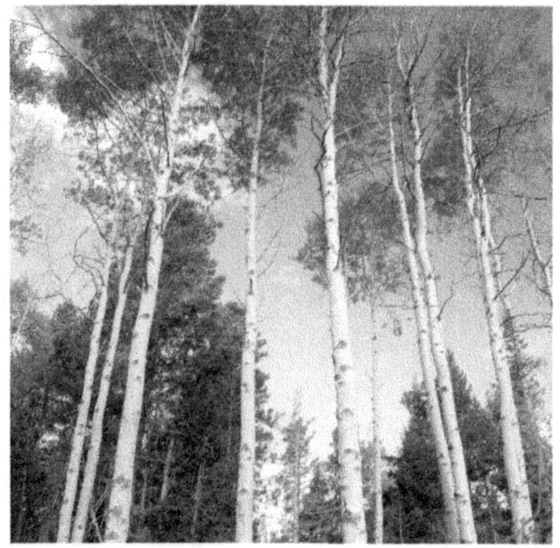

The inner bark or xylem is used in a tea to treat fevers, coughs and aches. It contains salicin, which is also found in willows and is the basic ingredient for aspirin.

Hawthorn Berry

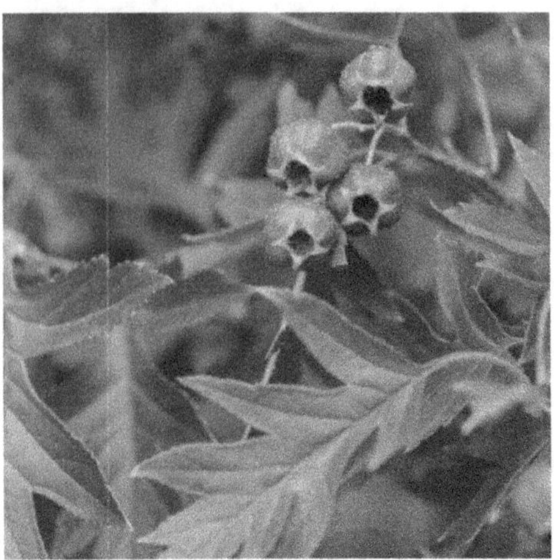

Natives used these berries in many ways, not only as a heart tonic but also for the management of many disorders, particularly concerning the feminine sphere.

Bee Pollen

When mixed with food it can increase energy, digestion and improve the immune system. If you are allergic to bee stings it is very likely that you are allergic to bee pollen.

Beeswax

Used as an ointment for burns and insect bites, including bee stings. Intended to be used externally only.

Blackberry

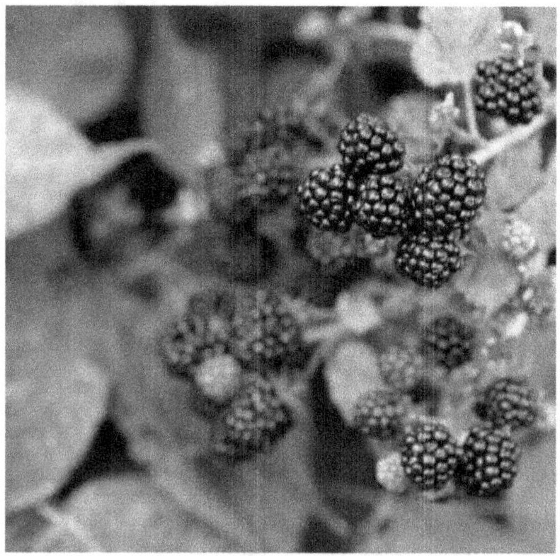

The root, bark and leaves when crushed and infused into a tea are used to treat diarrhea, reduce inflammation and stimulate metabolism. As a gargle it treats sore throats, mouth ulcers and inflammation of the gums.

Black Raspberry

The roots of this plant are crushed and used as a tea or boiled and chewed to relieve coughs, diarrhea and general intestinal discomfort.

Buckwheat

The seeds are used in soups and porridge as to lower blood pressure, helps with blood clotting and relieve diarrhea.

Cattail - typha

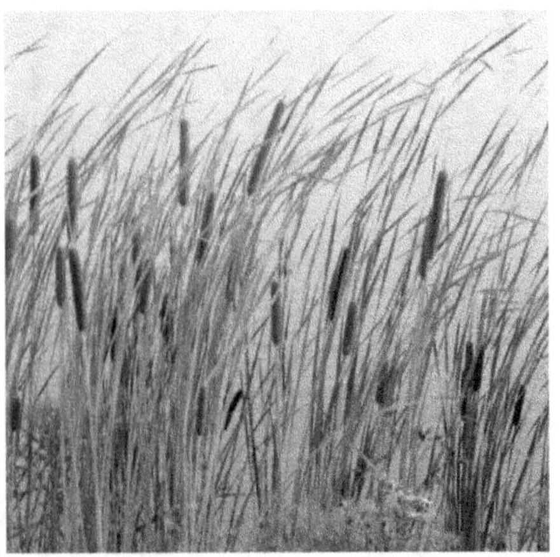

The Cherokee often ate cattails to speed up the body's healing process. Typically, Native Americans routinely harvested the typhus plant for use as bait, diaper material, and food. Typhus starch has even been found on Palaeolithic millstones dating back tens of thousands of years.

Cayenne

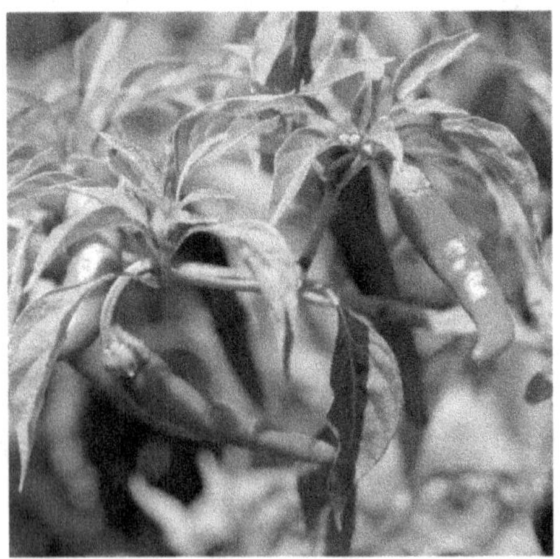

The pods are used as a pain reliever when taken with food or drunk in a tea. Also used for arthritis threats and digestive disorders. It is sometimes applied to wounds as a powder to increase blood flow and act as an antiseptic and anesthetic to numb the pain.

Chamomile

The leaves and flowers are used as a tea to treat intestinal problems and nausea.

Chokecherry

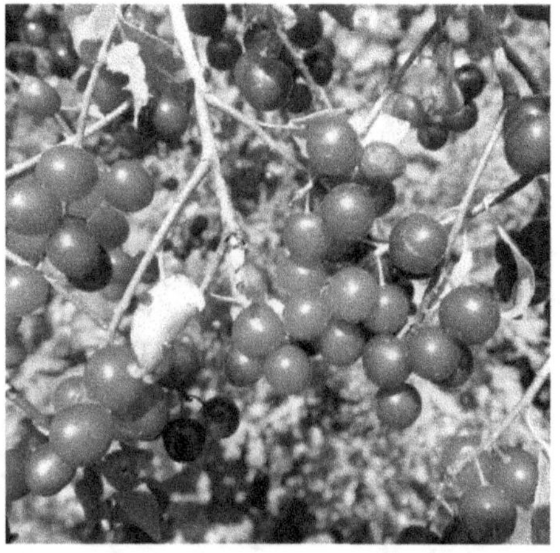

Considered by Native American tribes as an all-purpose medical treatment, the berries were pitted, dried and ground into a tea or poultice to treat a variety of ailments. These include coughs, colds, flu, nausea, inflammation and diarrhea. As an ointment or poultice it is used to treat burns and wounds. The seeds of chokecherry - much like apple seeds - are poisonous in high concentrations.

Chapparal

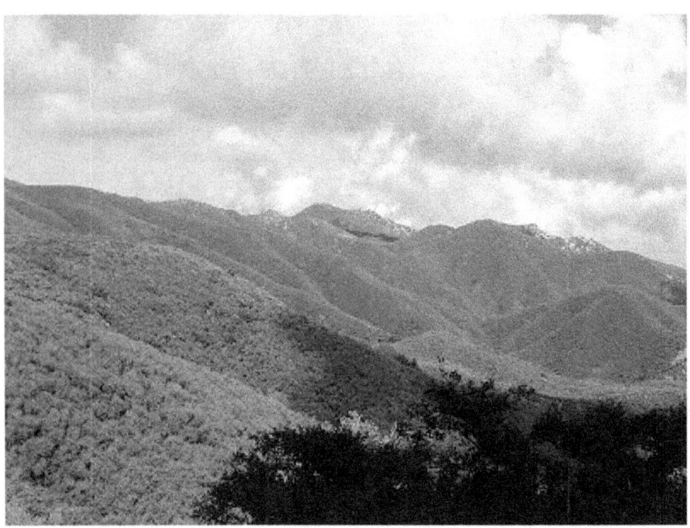

One of the favorite herbs of Native Americans, which was used in infusion form to treat symptoms of infectious origin.

Echinacea

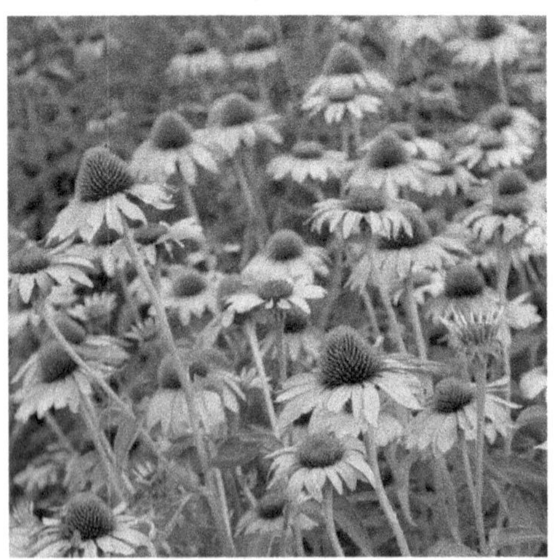

Also known as purple echinacea, this is a classic Native American medication that is used to strengthen the immune system, fight infection and fever. It is also used as an antiseptic and general treatment for colds, coughs and flu.

Edelberry – sambucus canadensis

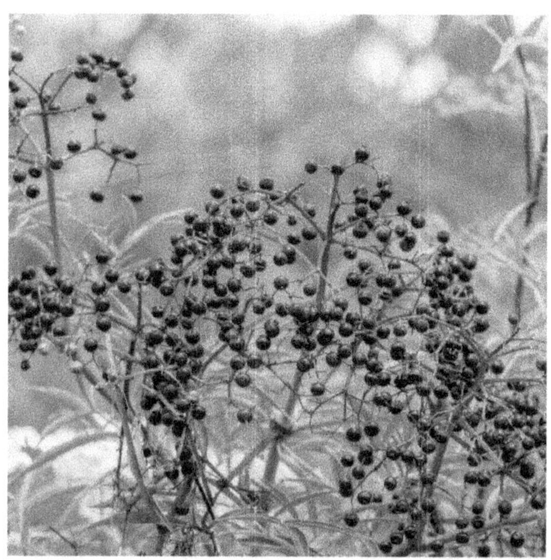

Wild American Elderberry (Sambucus canadensis) is a beautiful woody shrub, about 1 to 3.5 feet tall, with smooth yellow-gray twigs, bright green leaves arranged in a feather shape, and white pith.

Native Americans, who knew it well, used all parts of the plant, making tools from the branches and consuming the berries.

The plant contains many antioxidants that give the berries their red and purple color. Antioxidants help strengthen the immune system. In addition, elderberry extract contains anthocyanins that have anti-inflammatory properties, which can help in the treatment of arthritis and other chronic ailments. Historically, Native Americans used the plant in a tea to treat fever, coughs and pain.

Ephedra Trifurca

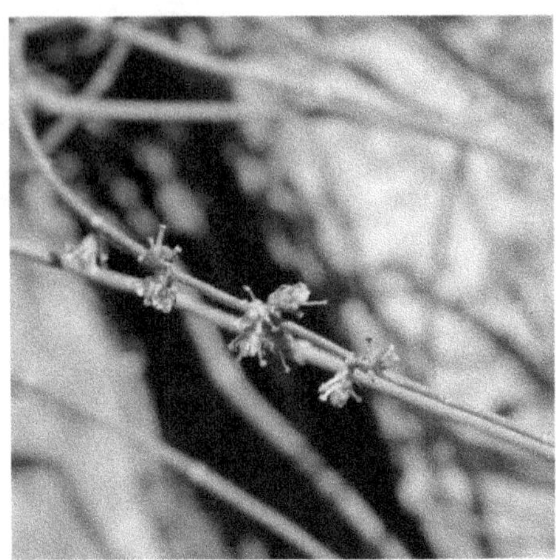

Ephedra trifurca goes by the common name of long jointed leaf fir and is most commonly found in Arizona. The seeds of Ephedra trifurca are in pairs and appear either black-red or grayish brown. Native Americans used trifurca for stomach problems, venereal diseases and kidney infections.

Mormon tea – ephedra nevadensis

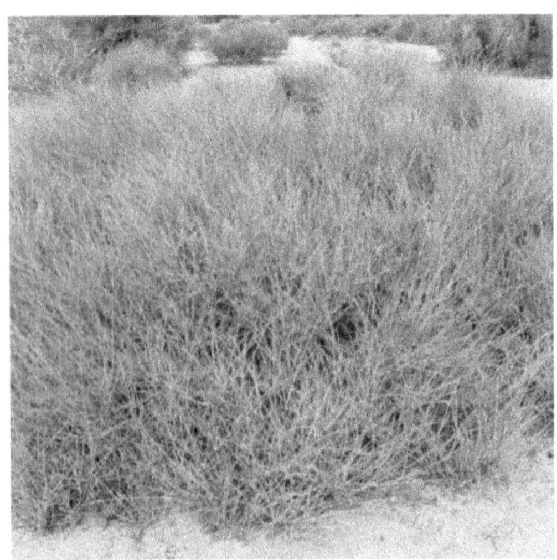

Mormon tea refers to several plants in the Ephedraceae family that are commonly found in the American Southwest and Mexico. A beverage made from the branched stems of the plant is called Mormon tea and was used as a folk remedy by indigenous groups and early American settlers. The herbal concoction was primarily used as a decongestant to relieve respiratory ailments such as asthma. In addition, the tea was used to treat urinary tract disorders and hypotension, and the stems of the plant were chewed as a remedy for sunburned lips.

Eucalyptus

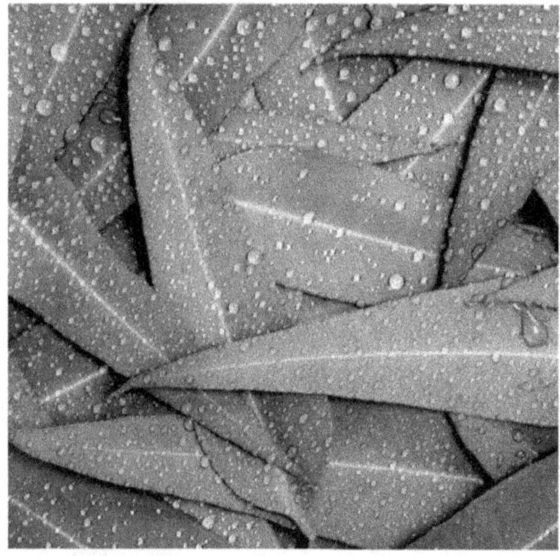

Oil from the leaves and roots is a common treatment when infused into a tea to treat coughs, sore throats, flu and fevers. It is used for this day as an ingredient in cough drops.

Fennel

A plant with a licorice flavor, this is used in a tea or chewed to relieve coughs, sore throats, digestion, offer relief to diarrhea and has been a general treatment for colds. It is also used as a poultice for the relief of eye and headaches.

Parthenium

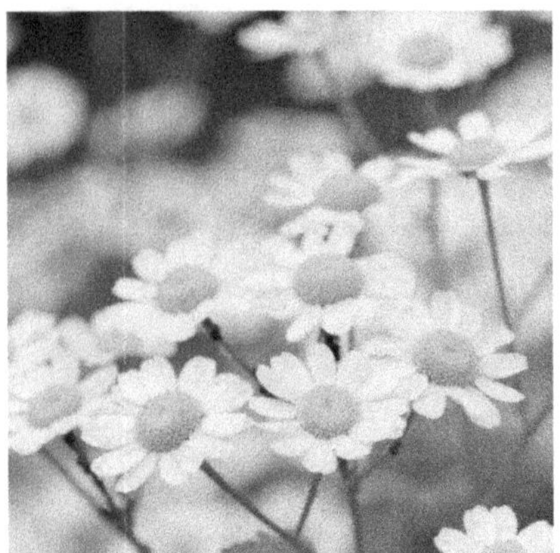

Use to this day as a natural relief for fever and headaches - including severe headaches such as migraines - it is also can be used for digestive problems, asthma and muscle and joint pain.

Poplar

The inner bark is used in herbal teas to treat fever, coughs, and pain. It contains salicin, which is also found in willows and is a basic ingredient in aspirin.

Red Elm

A natural calming agent popular with the Indians, who also used it to cleanse the body.

Feverwort

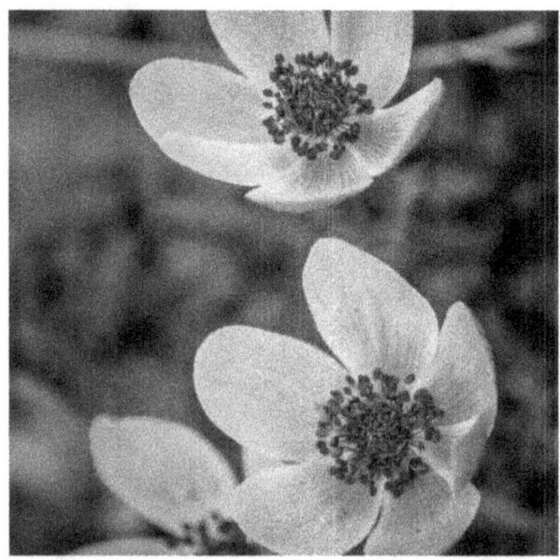

Another fever remedy that is also used for general pain, itching and joint stiffness. It can be ingested as a tea or chewed or crushed from a paste as an ointment or poultice.

Ginger

Another super plant in Native American medicine, the root was crushed and consumed with food, as a tea or ointment or poultice. Known for this day for its ability to aid digestive health, it is also anti-inflammatory, promotes circulation and can relieve colds, coughs and sniffles, as well as bronchitis and joint pain.

Ginseng

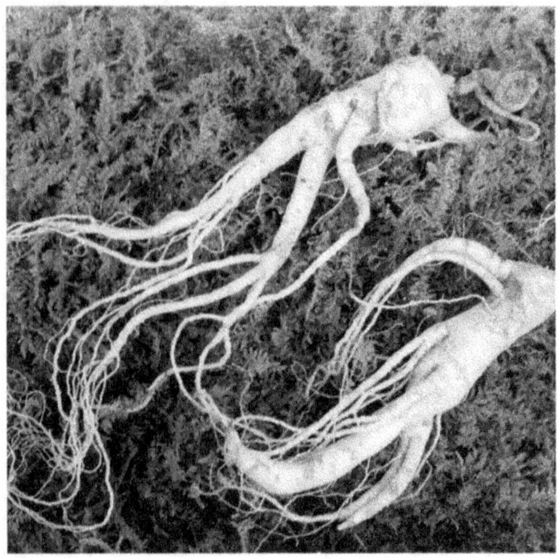

This is another contemporary herb that has a history that goes back through cultures for millennia. The roots have been used by Native Americans as a food additive, a tea and a poultice to treat fatigue, increase energy, improve the immune system and help with overall liver and lung function. The leaves and stems have also been used, but the root has the highest concentration of active ingredients.

Golden Rod - Asteracea

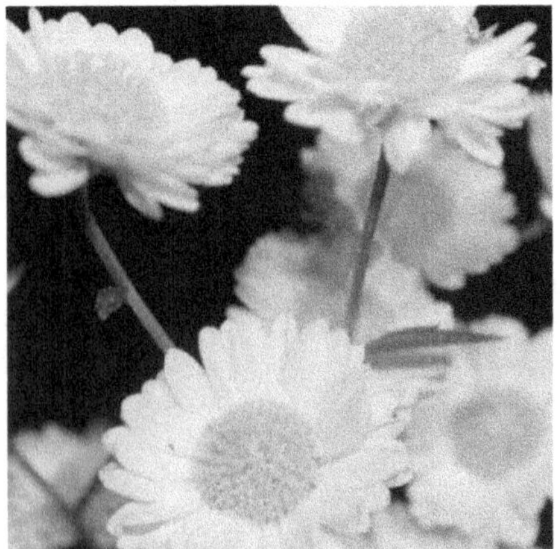

While these days it is considered a source of allergies and sneezing, it was actually considered another all-in-one medication by Native Americans. As a tea, an addition to food and a topical ointment, it is used to treat bronchitis

conditions and chest congestion to colds, flu, inflammation, sore throats and as an antiseptic for cuts and abrasions.

Honeysuckle

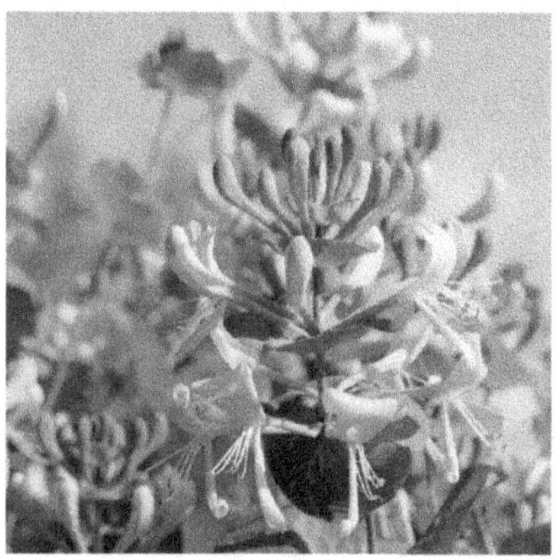

The berries, stems, flowers and leaves are used for topical treatment of bee stings and skin infections. As a tea, it is used to treat colds, headaches and sore throats. It also has anti-inflammatory properties.

Lady slipper orchid – cypripedium acaule

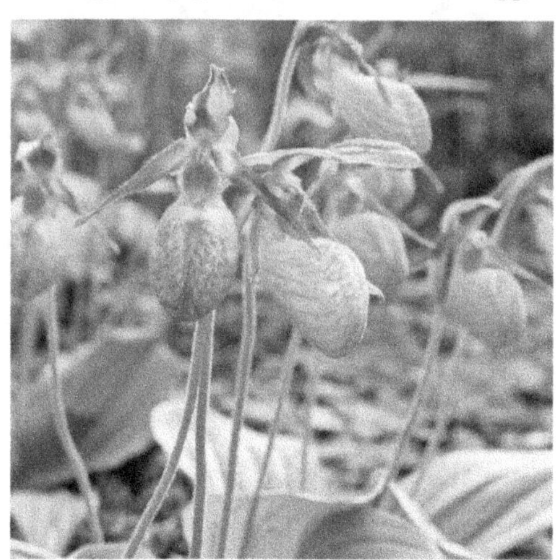

Pink Lady's Slipper (Cypripedium acaule Aiton) is a large, showy wildflower belonging to the orchid family. It blooms in the Adirondacks from late May to late June.

Pink Lady's Slippers were once used as a remedy for a variety of ailments, including nervousness, insomnia, kidney disorders and muscle spasms. Native Americans used an infusion of the roots for colds, fevers and urinary tract disorders.

Lavender

Lavender is traditionally used to calm the mind and relieve stress. One study reveals that lavender is a perfect remedy for insomnia, anxiety and depression, as well as headaches and fatigue.

Lobelia

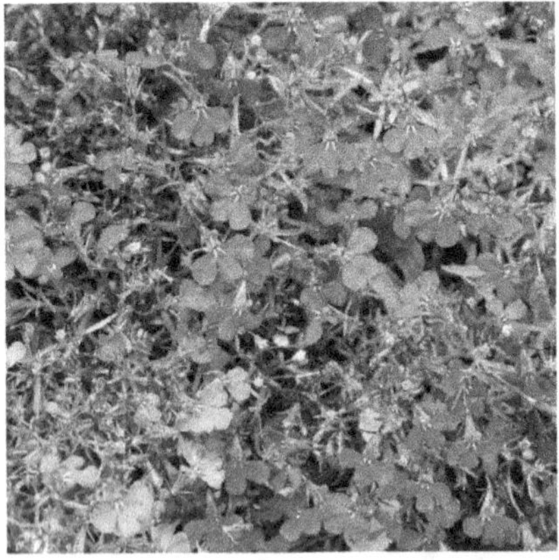

Plant similar to tobacco, it was highly considered by American Indians, who believed it had magical properties and for this reason they used it in spiritual rituals. It was successfully used for the treatment of syphilis and gonorrhea, two diseases brought by European settlers.

Polygala

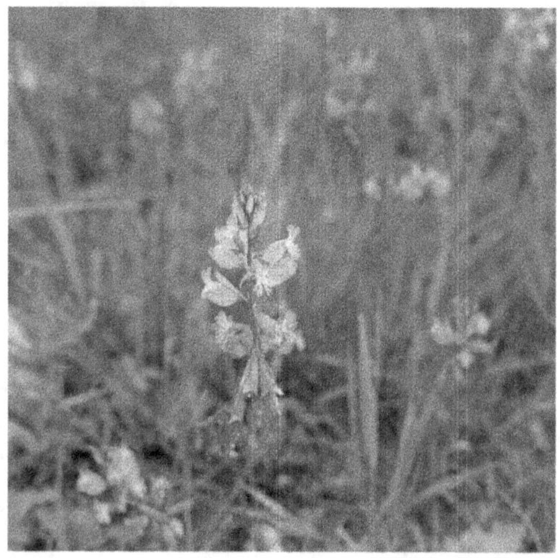

Also called "squaw root", it was used to counteract snake venom but, more generally, for the management of problems related to the female cycle.

Dioscorea root

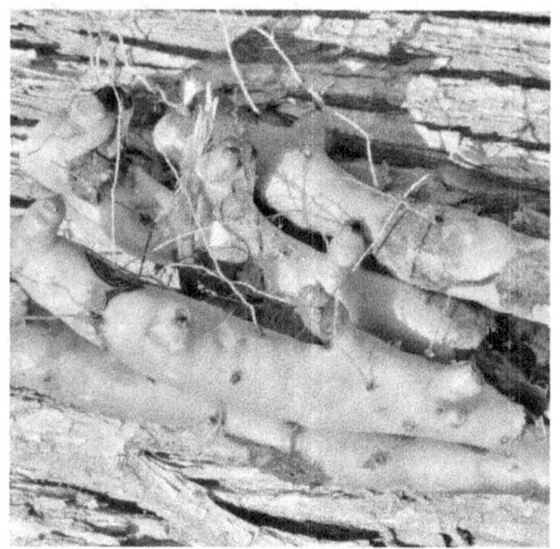

American Indians used it in moderate dosages in children because it has a soothing effect on colic, and in the elderly to relieve joint pain.

Oregon grape root

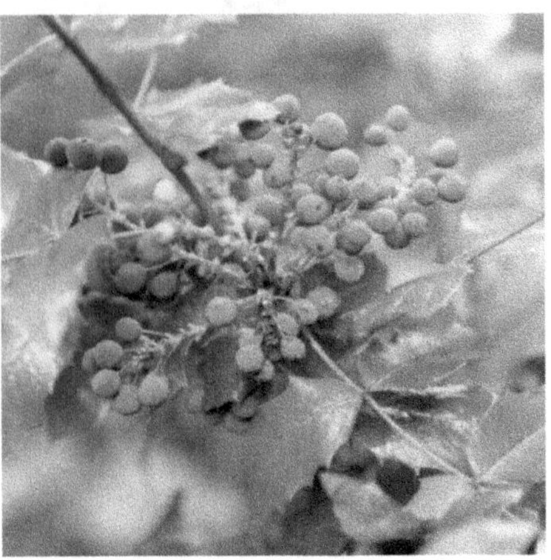

It was one of the most widely used herbs by Native Americans to treat wounds and abrasions.

Hops

As a tea that is used to treat digestive problems and often mixed with other herbs or plants, such as aloe, to soothe muscles. It is also used to soothe toothaches and sore throats.

Licorice

Roots and leaves can be used for coughs, colds, sore throats. The root can also be chewed to relieve toothache.

Verbasco

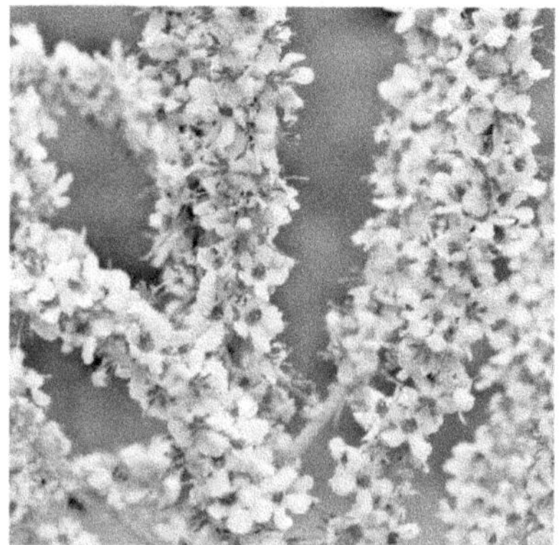

As an infusion in tea or added to a salad or other food, this is a plant that has been used by Native Americans to treat inflammation, coughing and lung congestion and general afflictions. It is quite common and likely to grow in your garden or somewhere nearby.

Passionflower

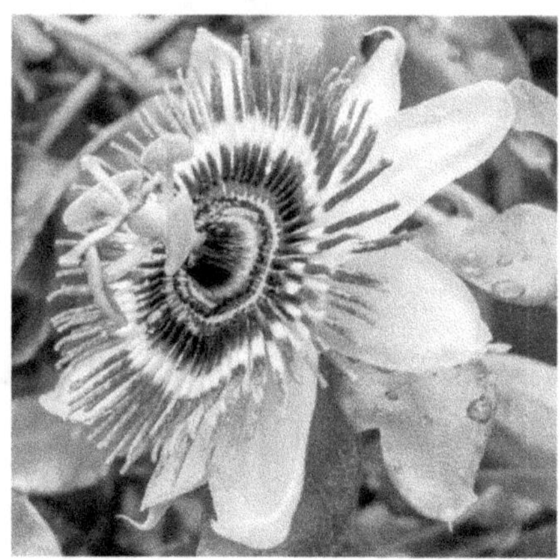

The leaves and roots are used to make a tea to treat anxiety and muscle pain. A poultice for skin injuries such as burns, insect bites and boils also can be made from passion flower.

Red clover

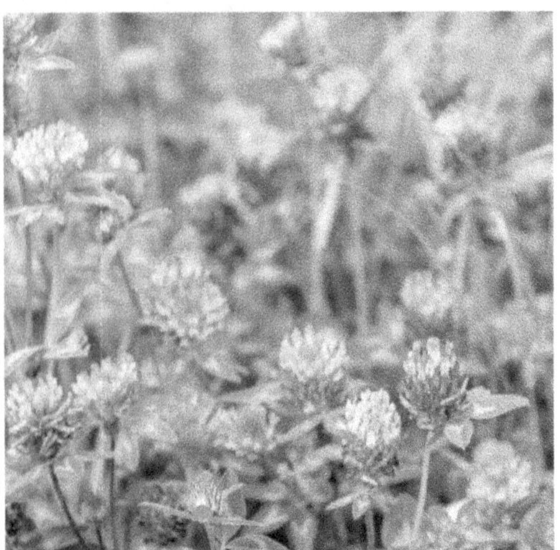

It grows everywhere and the flowers, leaves and roots are usually infused into a tea or are used for top feeding. It is used to manage inflammation, improve circulation and treat respiratory conditions.

Rosehip

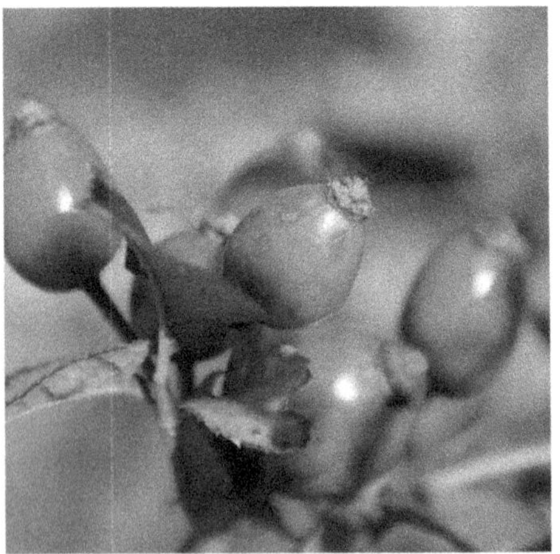

This is the red to orange berry that is the fruit of wild roses. It is already known to be a huge source of vitamin C and when consumed whole, mashed into a tea or added to food it is used to treat colds and coughs, intestinal difficulties, as an antiseptic and to treat inflammation.

Rosemary

A member of the pine family and used in food products and as a tea to treat muscle pain, improve circulation and as a general cleanser for the metabolism.

Spearmint

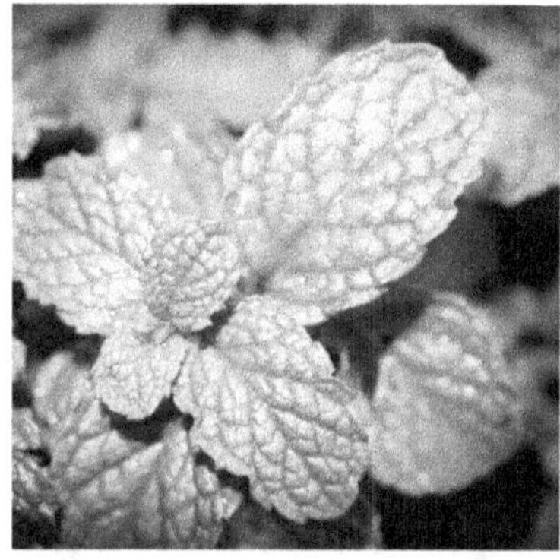

Machines constantly by Native American tribes to treat coughs, colds, breathing difficulties and as a cure for diarrhea and a stimulant for blood circulation.

Valerian

The root as an infusion in a tea relieves muscle aches, pain and is said to have a calming effect.

Yarrow – achillea millefolium

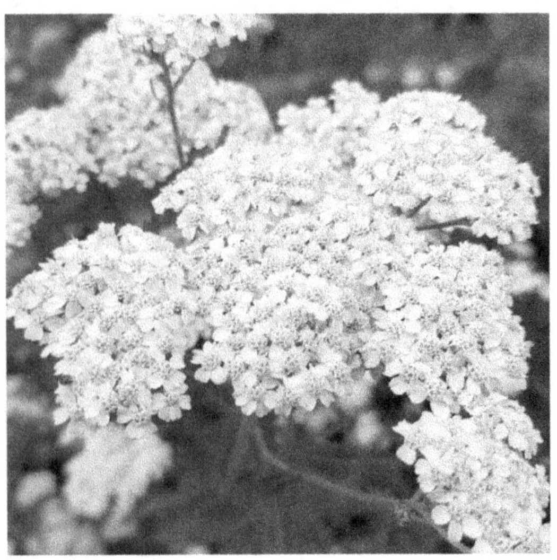

Native Americans used the plant in topical applications for wounds, abrasions, hematomas, eczema, muscle aches, rashes and earaches. Internally it was used as a remedy for digestive disorders (slow or weak digestion) sense of malaise and febrile conditions (both internally and as fumigations with burnt flowers). The leaf and flowers were official drugs in the American Pharmacopoeia from 1863 to 1882, for tonic, stimulant, and emmenagogue use.

Native Americans of the Menomini tribe used the plant to treat fevers (hot infusion of the leaves), while the flowering tops were used as a rub for eczema. The leaves were used as a poultice for children's skin rash.

White Pine

Ubiquitous and the needles and inner bark can be infused into a tea. Used as a standard treatment for respiratory distress and chest congestion.

Witch hazel – hamamelis virginiana

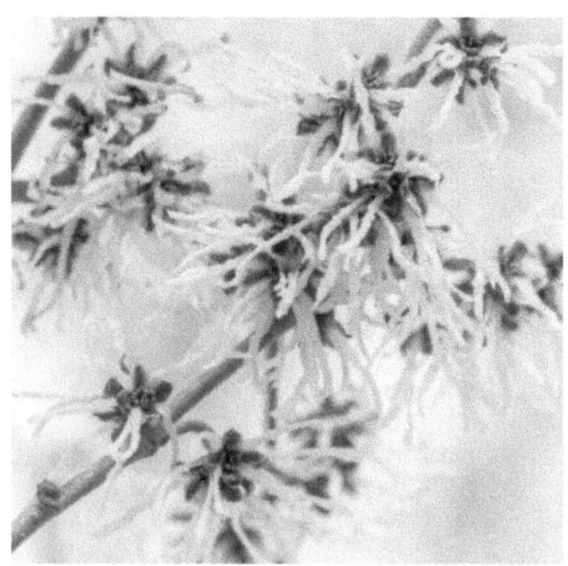

Native Americans had already discovered the astringent and vasoconstrictive properties of Witch Hazel: they applied on bleeding wounds the liquid obtained by boiling twigs in water for a long time, and this quickly stopped bleeding and facilitated the healing of the wound. This fact was used by the "sorcerers-herbalists" as magic to heal wounds of warriors, and therefore Hamamelis was considered a magical plant.

Perhaps learning of these beliefs, early American settlers gave it the name Witch-hazel, which means "witch-hazel," and in the United States to this day Witch Hazel water is called by that name.

Witch hazel branches are very flexible and it seems dowsers drew from them saplings they considered particularly sensitive to find sources of underground waters, reinforcing the beliefs about "magical" properties attributed to this plant.

The chemical composition of this plant is very complex, but the most interesting substances from a physiotherapeutic point of view are flavonoids, phenols, mucilages, essential oil, tannins, gallic acid, which have an astringent venous, hemostatic, antihemorrhagic, antiphlogistic and decongestant activity, which confirms the traditional popular use of Witch Hazel.

Herbal Remedies

Remedy against Scurvy

The first contact with Indian medicine dates back to 1535 when the members of the naval crew led by the French explorer Jacques Cartier began to die of scurvy, a disease caused by a massive deficiency of vitamin C in the body and that manifests itself with bleeding sores. Faced with the dramatic situation, the captain played the last card: he sent one of his sailors, sick but still strong, in search of an unexpected help.

After a few days the man came back healed: the man was lucky to find a tribe of Native Americans who cured him with remedies based on pine and juniper, whose extracts of bark and leaves were applied to the wounds. The sailor brought the cure to the ship and the crew was saved.

Remedies to purify the environment and the person

The natives were known for their purification practices, not only of the person but also of the environment. For this purpose they used to burn sprigs of sacred plants that had the ability to eliminate and remove stagnant and negative energies, smudges, the equivalent of our incense, made with dried sprigs of sacred plants such as White Sage, Palo santo, Cedar, and Yerba santa.

They were also burned during religious ceremonies or propitiatory rites to protect the person from any energetic obstacles. Among the most known shamanic rituals there was also the sweat lodge (Inipi in the native language of North America, Temazcal for Mayans) a sacred rite which had the symbolic purpose of experiencing the return to the belly of Mother Earth, in order to get rid of toxins that pollute body, mind and spirit and that cause disease on different levels, through a steam bath.

The rite included the construction of the hut, which has at its center a hole dug in the ground where hot stones are placed on which water is sprayed, releasing, in this way, steam. During the ceremony, participants sang songs and prayers until the conclusion of the ritual, when it was customary to smoke the sacred pipe.

How to purify the house with the Native American technique.

Occasionally it is a good idea to purify the house. It is especially important to do this after a crowded gathering, a family bereavement, a visit from an unwanted guest, an argument, or once a year during spring cleaning.

To purify your entire home, fumigate each room with sage sticks or burn incense in each room, keeping the windows open. Negative energies will escape to the outside, where they will dissolve.

Another method to purify a house is to use a large iron pan in which to burn salt (salt has a strong purifying power; a Celtic method to keep negative energies away from the outside is to pour salt around the foundations of the house) and with which to walk around the house fumigating each room. It can also help to light white or purple candles and use aromatic oils, incense or myrrh.

Natural echinacea decoction

Echinacea herbal tea is obtained from the dried and shredded plant and in particular from its root which is then put inside sachets or sold in bulk for the preparation of herbal tea. In the preparation of herbal tea it is not possible to quantify and standardize the percentage of active substances and therefore it could be little or too concentrated. It is however suggested the use of a maximum of 2 cups of decoction per day and for a maximum time of 2 consecutive weeks. Echinacea decoction is prepared by adding one tablespoon of dried echinacea root in 200 ml of cold water. This is brought to a boil and kept for 5 minutes, then subsequently removed from the heat and left to steep for another 10 minutes. It is filtered and drunk by adding honey, lemon juice or other natural sweeteners to taste.

Echinacea decoction is useful both for external use for compresses and washes on skin that has scars, dermatitis, irritation, inflammation, canker sores or other skin problems. It brings with it immunostimulant, anti-inflammatory, protective, healing properties thus managing to create a suitable environment that accelerates the regeneration of epithelial tissues and soothes infections. Moreover this decoction of echinacea is used for all the problems we previously mentioned and in particular for cough, cold, sore throat and flu.

Recipe with echinacea and rose hip

With the same preparation of the decoction of echinacea we can make it and add a half spoonful of rosehip berries. Remember to let the decoction rest for at least 10 minutes in order to allow all the active principles to come out from the herbs and to be poured in the herbal tea. These two official plants are enhanced because to the properties of echinacea are added those of dog rose, very rich in vitamin C, helps to strengthen the immune system, fight against infections and relieve respiratory diseases.

Recipe with echinacea and altea roots

Another formulation is the decoction of echinacea roots and marshmallow roots. The preparation remains the same as decoction with one level tablespoon of echinacea and one level tablespoon of marshmallow. This decoction can be used externally with compresses and washes to aid in the healing and regeneration of the epidermis when there are skin problems. Due to the presence of its mucilage, marshmallow adds the properties of emollient, soothing and inflammatory to those of echinacea. In addition to external use, drinking the decoction of echinacea and altea also helps the mucous membranes of the gastrointestinal tract and strengthens the immune system.

Smudge Stick or Shamanic Incense

Smudges, or smudge sticks are natural incense, characteristic of the culture of shamans and indigenous peoples. They are typically associated to the tradition of South American Indians, although they are widespread in many other areas of the world, for example in Africa, where they are part of the purification rituals performed by Sufis.

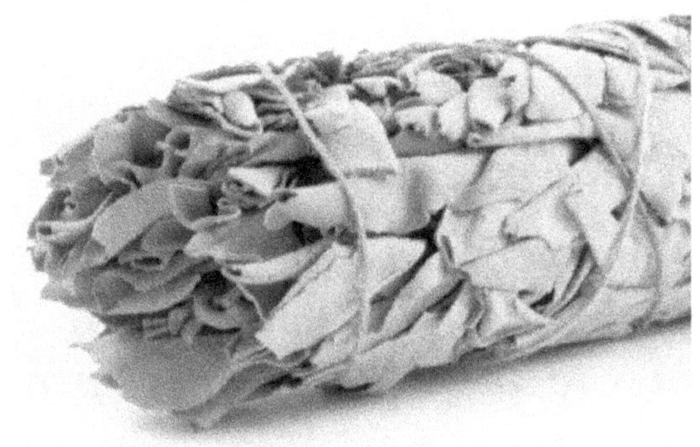

Smudge sticks are in fact incenses made from dried herbs and flowers, and are used to purify environments, people or objects from negative energies, combining the release of aromas and essential oils through combustion, to the beneficial and therapeutic properties of plants, conveyed through fumigation: smudging means burning herbs and incense.

Smoking is a very important element in shamanic spiritual purification rituals, and the use of dried plants as incense in religious ceremonies and healing of the sick is thousands of years old.

To date, smudging is best known for its association with purification rituals and indigenous spiritual religious ceremonies, in which the smoke obtained from burning smudges is used to rid environments, people and things of negative thoughts and energies.

As we mentioned, smudge is a type of natural incense that is traditionally used in shamanic purification rituals.

Although the practice of smudging is at a more spiritual level than physical, in addition to the mystical dimension these incenses allow you to enjoy the many properties of plants that are used within them: from plants with relaxing and calming effect, such as lavender, herbs that improve concentration and focus, even plants with antibacterial effect, the smudge sticks do not necessarily have to be used within religious ceremonies but can be burned to release essential oils from the countless benefits to mind and body.

In shamanic purification rituals smudges are used to free places, objects and people from negative energies: it will often happen to you to enter a room and feel a heavy air, an unpleasant feeling, which can be associated with a bad energy. In indigenous American peoples smudge sticks are used in rituals and religious ceremonies of purification of environments, people or objects with which they come into contact. In shamanic culture smoking has a very important symbolic value, because according to the belief it would create a way of communication with the realm of energies and spirituality. In indigenous rituals the smoke of sweetgrass, cedar, white sage and tobacco is generally used to free a person, room or object from negative thoughts, spirits or energies.

Smudging is also used for meditation in different tribes and cultures around the world since ancient times, as according to tradition through purification by smoke released from plants you can move between the physical and spiritual world. Today shamanic incenses are very popular in the West as well, and they are used in rituals and purification practices inspired by shamanic traditions.

How to prepare a Smudge Stick?

Smudge sticks can be bought ready-made, or prepared at home in case you have aromatic herbs and flowers: making a do-it-yourself smudge stick is very simple, and allows you to use your favorite herbs and aromas, combining them to enjoy their scents and properties.

To make a smudge stick it is necessary to use fresh plants, leaves and flowers, as by using already dried herbs you would risk to break them during the binding. It is therefore necessary to collect the plants, making sure to collect them in their balsamic time, the period when the content of essential oils in the plant is higher and they are more ready to give their power of purification and protection. With the fumigation, in fact, are going to release the essential oils of herbs, which through breathing allow you to enjoy the properties attributed to them. The balsamic time varies from plant to plant, but often falls in the summer months: it is however preferable, in case you decide to combine more plants in a single smudge stick, to choose herbs that have the same balsamic time.

To prepare smudge sticks it is possible to use different plants and flowers, the most used are sage, rosemary, lavender, cedar, laurel and thyme, but you can choose your favorite aromas, and choose to prepare smudges with only one type of plant, in order to enjoy its single properties, or combine them in a scented mix, according to the type of purification you want to do.

For the smudges you will need sprigs of about 10-20 cm in length (depending on the desired length). You can also use flower petals or leaves, to embellish your bundles of incense, but you will have to be very careful in tying them, as they may slip away from the wire: in this regard are preferred the wider petals such as rose petals, which can be wrapped around the bundle of herbs.

You can also place pieces of bark inside the twigs, such as holy palm tree logs, or incense grains or resins, such as myrrh grains, to create even more unique combinations of scents and properties for your purification rituals. You can discover the different types of incense grains in Terza Luna's online shop and choose from a variety of flavors and properties.

After collecting the herbs and cut the twigs so that they are more or less all of the same length join them, keeping them in the same direction, in a small bundle, which will be tied using a natural cotton thread or a string.

To tie the smudge, twist the twine in a spiral along the length of the bundle of herbs, from the bottom to the top, and then back out, making a double loop at the base and stopping the stick with a knot, creating a loop that will allow you to hang your smudge for drying. Be sure to tie the twigs carefully, to prevent any leaves from escaping the knot.

At this point your smudge is ready and will need to be left to dry for use. Hang it using the loop you created with the wire: this will allow the essential oils to descend and concentrate in the end of the smudge, which is the part that is normally burned.

How to Use the Smudge Stick?

Once the smudge stick is dried it can be burned for purification rituals. As we have seen smudging is a very ancient practice, aimed at purifying environments, people and things from negative energies. They can be used for meditation, before going to sleep, or simply to perfume a room and improve breathing. Using certain plants with antibacterial and antiviral action can also purify environments.

In order to use smudge sticks it will be enough to light with a match or a lighter the end of the bundle of herbs, extinguishing the flame immediately. The bundle of herbs will still continue to burn, releasing a smoke that will spread in the environment.

Room Purification

To use the smudge in room purification make sure to close the windows so that the smoke stays inside the room. You can let the smudge burn in a stone container, or move around the room, always in a clockwise direction, making sure to linger longer in the most lived-in parts of the room, such as a table, or a bed, without forgetting the corners. Open the windows, to let out the smoke along with the negative energies.

Purification of the Person

For purification of the body, light the smudge stick in the same way, extinguish it and move it around the body, starting from the head, breathing in the smoke deeply, passing around the chest and shoulders, to the legs, spreading the smoke with the hands or a feather.

Sacred plants of the four directions

EAST

The herbs associated with the East direction are pine, sage and tobacco.

Tobacco: It is and was used to honour the ancestors invoking their wisdom in order to decide on important issues of one's life or the life of the tribe.

Pine: This plant is used to cleanse the aura, obtain fertility and peace of mind. There are many American Indians who use it in their homes, because it is thought to be a good guardian, being of the evergreen family so it never dies and always remains vigilant.

SOUTH

The sacred herbs associated with the direction of the South that are used in prayers, are the cedar and copal.

Cedar: It is used to protect oneself or one's loved ones from evil in a general sense, it is connected to the sun and serves to attract new life.

Copal: It is used specifically in ceremonies of the South-West direction to facilitate the fluidity of the energies that are moved.

WEST

The sacred herbs used for this direction are sage, mugwort and willow.

Sage: Belongs to the sacred herbs par excellence that purify, strengthen and protect in addition to the fact that it is one of the herbs that can defeat even the most serious diseases and disorders from which it takes its name (salvia: salvis = life saver), destroys and removes the dark forces and in fact it is one of the most widely used magical Indian herbs in rituals, sometimes it is also used for sacred rites directed to the direction of the East, but all its characteristics are focused on the qualities of the West.

Mugwort: This sacred herb is used because it helps in visions and because it makes it easier to have lucid and clear dreams as well as to prophesy.

Willow: According to several legends this plant represents the unconscious part of people, which brings a renewal of their life after death.

NORTH

The most sacred grass to the north direction, is represented by the sweet grass which means "grandmother's hair", in fact this white "hair" would correspond to the symbol of experience and wisdom generated by the experiences made in life.

Native American Beverages

Since ever primitive people and not only American Indians tried to flavor the water they drank in order to get over the boredom of the lack of taste or maybe even if unconsciously they were looking for a way to heal or keep healthy thanks to aromatic herbs.

Drinks could be drunk both cold and hot as well as being fermented in order to give the alcoholic component to the beverage even though among American Indians the alcohol by volume has always been kept low in order to prevent unsuitable behaviors in social life, just like they discovered at their own expense with the so called "fire water" which was nothing else than a grappa or a very strong derivative that obscured the mind releasing in natives the normal inhibitory brakes.

Native American Potions

ACCORD (Quercus)

Acorn shells were roasted well, then put in water to boil for 15 minutes, then strained and served as a coffee.

BEARBERRY (Bearberry)

Bearberry, a low evergreen shrub that prefers acidic soils; dried leaves are used to make an astringent tea with a pleasantly tart flavor, useful for settling the stomach. One teaspoon per cup, steeping in boiling water for 15 min.

BETULLE

Tree from which many Tribes derive sap in Spring to make a fresh and nutritious drink, it is still used for "Birch Beer" and for vinegars.

BLUE COTTOSH (Indian name) SQUAW

The bluish seeds are roasted, ground and then boiled, with them an excellent coffee is made. It is used 1 teaspoon per cup, boiling them slowly for 15 minutes, then filter and serve.

DMANY (Cunila Origanoides) Native perennial plant, it was used for hot drinks by many Indian Tribes to treat colds. One tablespoon of leaves per cup infused for 15 minutes.

ELDEBERRY (Elderberry, Sambucas canadiensis)

One teaspoon of flowers to grind for 15 min. in hot water gives an excellent herbal tea. The flowers can be added to tea to give more flavor. From the red-purple berries boiled, a sweet syrup is obtained which was used as an elixir or diluted with water to make a delicious fruit drink.

LIFE EVERLASNG (Eternal Life)

Plant very appreciated by Native Americans. The whole plant, including flowers, can be dried in order to obtain a pleasant beverage, similar to a light tea. 2 litres of boiling water, 1 pinch of Life Everlasting, infuse for 15 minutes.

Herbal Preparation

Herbal teas, decoctions and infusions have remarkable therapeutic virtues and knowing how to prepare them is fundamental to acquire all their beneficial properties.

Infusions, decoctions and tisanes are the officinal preparations that can be easily made at home and they have been used for centuries to treat many diseases and disorders. The term "officinal" derives from Latin and indicates the plants which were used in the apothecary's store (the ancient pharmacist), which was called workshop. Therefore, medicinal plants are defined as those plants which contain in one of their parts, in one of their organs (roots, barks, seeds, buds, leaves, flowers, fruits), some substances, called active principles, which can be used for therapeutic purposes.

Drug means the part of the plant used.

To prepare a therapeutic herbal tea are used more vegetable drugs that, "are mixtures of vegetable drugs, intended for the preparation of herbal teas, which are divided into fragments of a size suitable for carrying out the preparations, separated by rags from the fine powder, which must be discarded". Vegetable drugs, "must be chosen and cleaned with care and can be used whole or conveniently reduced in fragments of a size suitable for the execution of the preparation".

Herbal teas are undoubtedly useful and allow even non-experts of phytotherapy, whether doctors or patients, to gradually become familiar with medicinal plants.

Therapeutic herbal teas (infusions and decoctions) are undoubtedly the most used mode of administration by Native Americans. Therapeutic herbal teas have the following advantages compared to other officinal forms:

- *easy absorption of active principles*

- *rapidity of action of the absorbed active principles*
- *possibility to modify the ingredients from time to time*

On the contrary, decoctions have the following disadvantages

- *more time dedicated to the preparation*
- *often unpleasant smell and taste that sometimes the decoction can assume*

It is recommended the use of decoctions especially in acute pathologies, in which the speed of absorption of active principles and therefore their rapidity of action are important and determinant elements for the effectiveness of therapy. The effectiveness of a herbal tea depends by the way it is prepared, by respecting the doses, the infusion or decoction time and the dosage. It is very important that the preparation of a therapeutic herbal tea is done according to precise rules codified since millennia in order to exalt the effectiveness and the therapeutic action of the officinal plants present in it.

How to prepare a herbal tea

Herbal teas are prepared by maceration, by digestion, by infusion, by decoction, using drinking water and, before being used, they are decanted or, if necessary, filtered through absorbent cotton or gauze".

Infusion

Let's remember infusion is prepared by pouring water at boiling temperature on the drugs, reduced to a suitable level of subdivision, and then leaving them in contact with water for a more or less long time. After complete cooling it is necessary to filter through absorbent cotton or gauze and then bring the filtrate to the prescribed mass with hot water with which the residue and the filter are washed.

The infusion method is used when the active ingredients are volatile (essential oils) or alterable by intense and prolonged heat. Generally infusions are practiced on drugs with delicate tissue such as flowers, buds, leaves. When, however, the infusion is prepared with leathery leaves, for example of Arctostaphylos uva-ursi (Bearberry) or Laurus nobilis (Laurel), or with compact drugs (roots, rhizomes, seeds) it is advisable to precede the infusion a sufficiently long maceration.

The infusion, therefore, is obtained by pouring a certain quantity of water at boiling temperature, in a container where there are already the drugs previously minced or chopped; it is left to macerate everything in a covered container, for an appropriate time, then it is filtered and the residual is compressed. This is an excellent method when using earthenware or porcelain containers (which keep the heat for a long time) properly heated by boiling some water which is obviously to be thrown away before using the container.

The average drug/water ratio is about 3-5 grams of drug every 100 ml of water, with some exceptions: the infusion of Carimi carvi (Caraway) and Anethum graveolens (Dill) fruits is 0.6-0.8 g/100 ml. The time of contact between drugs and water determines color, taste and activity of the therapeutic herbal tea, which can be regulated by everyone according to their own tastes and needs. The posology is on average of one cup 3-4 times a day. The average infusion time of the various drugs is of 7-10 minutes, however it can be prolonged to 15-20 minutes according to the type of drugs used and the active principles to be extracted.

A shorter extraction time, 2-3 minutes, allows the preparation of a not therapeutic herbal tea, but only pleasing as it releases only the aromatic, volatile and thermolabile active principles and not the active principles which are slow to solubilize. According to the chemical nature of the active principles to be extracted from drugs, it is appropriate to use some tricks in order to improve the efficiency of extraction.

The infusion, being an extemporaneous preparation, should be consumed soon after its preparation, hot or lukewarm, never boiling or cold. It can be sweetened or not with honey, fructose, cane sugar.

Decoction

Decoction is obtained by boiling in water more drugs from which one wants to extract the active principles. Decoction is a violent process, such as to destroy some active principles and denature organic components. Decoctions are "liquid preparations obtained, extemporaneously, by boiling in water the drugs properly pulverized, from which one wants to extract the active principles. The corresponding operation is called decoction and it is never applied to drugs containing volatile active principles. Usually five parts of drugs are used to prepare 100 parts of decoction.

Decoction is suitable for compact and lignified or otherwise leathery drugs such as:

- the wood of Santalum album (Sandalwood)

- barks of *Aesculus hyppocastanum* (Horse chestnut), *Piscidia erythrina* (Piscidia), *Rhamnus purshiana* (Cascara sagrada)
- the roots of *Althaea officinalis* (Altea), *Arctium lappa* (Burdock), *Echinacea purpurea* (Echinacea), *Glycyrrhiza glabra* (Licorice), *Juglans regia* (Walnut), *Ononis spinosa* (Ononide), *Urtica dioica* (Nettle), *Rheum officinale* (Rhubarb), *Ruscus aculeatus* (Butcher's Broom), *Taraxacum officinale* (Dandelion);
- the seeds of *Sylibum marianum* (Milk Thistle).

But it also suits those non-hard drugs such as:

- the leaves of *Cynara scolymus* (Artichoke), *Combretum micranthum* (Combreto), *Gingko-biloba* (Gingko), *Ilex paraguariensis* (Maté), *Juglans regia* (Walnut), *Malva sylvestris* (Mallow), *Urtica dioica* (Nettle), *Vaccinium myrtillus* (Bilberry), *Verbascum thapsus* (Mullein), *Vinca minor* (Periwinkle)
- cauliculi of *Equisetum arvense* (Horsetail)
- bulbs of *Allium cepa* (Onion)
- the peel of *Solanum melongena* (Eggplant)
- the thallus of *Cetraria Islandica* (Icelandic Lichen), *Fucus vesiculosus* (Sea Owl)
- fruits of *Crataegus monogyna* (Hawthorn), *Physalis alkekengi* (Alchechengi), *Sorbus domesticus* (Rowan)
- styles of the female flowers of *Zea mays* (Corn)

These drugs only after a prolonged action of heat release to the solvent their active principles, stable to heat, sufficiently hydrophilic but difficult to solubilize, such as tannins, many alkaloids, triterpenes, flavonoids.

It is good practice to crush, grind or pulverize drugs before using them, in order to facilitate water in its work of extraction of active principles.

The decoction of barks, roots, woods, involves a boiling time from 6 to 30 minutes, according to the hardness of the drug and a subsequent infusion period of not less than 5-10 minutes, in order to favor the exit of the active principles from the vegetal cells and their passage in the water. In case of particularly hard drugs it is appropriate to grind them and to macerate them for some hours, taking care to avoid fermentation, which could hydrolyse glycosidic bonds and therefore make some active principles less assimilable. For non-hard drugs 5-10 minutes of boiling are enough.

For decoctions the average drug/water ratio is about 3-5 g of drugs per 100 ml of water. The dosage is always one cup 2-3 times a day. Also in decoctions the contact time between drug and water determines color, taste and activity.

Decoction is generally drunk during the day, before meals in order to favor its absorption. In case the decoction contains substances having irritating effects on the digestive system, it should always be consumed after meals, as well as it should always be consumed after meals by patients having gastric or intestinal irritations.

How to prepare a herbal tea with hot extraction

Once we have chosen the accessories and the objects for herbal teas that we like the most, the right ingredients, we can proceed to the preparation of the perfect herbal tea.

Fill the filter - disposable sachets or infusers - with the mix of herbs, spices and fruits that you like the most

Insert the filter in the cup

Bring water to a boil in a herbal tea kettle

Pour the boiling water into the cup with the filter inside

Cover with a cloth or a lid

Wait for about 10 minutes

Remove the filter - which can be used for a second and even third infusion

Once slightly cooled down we can consume our herbal tea or infusion while enjoying its benefits, its warmth and its taste.

How to make herbal tea with cold extraction
There are very fresh and delicious cold infusions prepared with the Cold Brew method.

Let's see how to do it:

- Fill the filter with your favorite herbal tea or tea
- Fill a pitcher with cold or room temperature water
- Immerse the filter in the water and cover with a lid or cloth
- Refrigerate for 3 to 6 hours
- Remove the filter and store in the refrigerator

By cold-pressing your herbal teas and infusions, not only will you be able to enjoy a refreshing and thirst-quenching drink, but you will also be able to enjoy all the properties that the chosen herbal tea possesses, just like a normal hot herbal tea. In addition, however, you can keep your herbal tea cold for up to 7 days, as long as you maintain the cold chain, without affecting either the taste or the organoleptic properties of the infusion.

Poultice

To prepare an abdominal poultice, you must pour natural cold water into a ceramic, glass or wooden bowl (never use plastic or metal containers) and then add the granular clay, until it covers the surface of the water. This preparation is allowed to stand until the clay has absorbed all the water. After mixing well with a wooden ladle, a soft, smooth, homogeneous and fluid paste is obtained.

The preparation with a thickness of about one centimeter must then be spread on a wrapping paper. A gauze is then spread over the clay and applied directly and gently to the abdomen, taking care to cover it well from side to side. Afterwards the preparation is covered with a cotton cloth and a woollen cover that will wrap well the abdomen of the subject under treatment, being careful not to leave air pockets. If the clay is kept all night long, in the morning the painful or inflammatory condition will be greatly attenuated thanks to the thermo-absorbing power of this material.

If after two-three hours from the application the clay should still be soft and wet, it means that the part of the body treated is cold and does not react to the poultice: in this case it is recommended to reduce the thickness. On the contrary, if the clay tends to dry and dry too quickly, it means that the treated part is very hot and therefore it is necessary to increase the thickness. In any case, at the time of removal, the clay must be dry enough to be crumbled.

The poultice should always be performed cold on the intact skin of a warm body. Therefore, do not do it when you feel very cold, for example if you have just returned home in winter or if you have a cold. The only exception is when applying it to the kidneys, for which case the poultice must be prepared with warm water.

Essential Oils

It is a liquid substance with an oily aspect, of variable color according to the plant used, extremely powerful, volatile and scented. It is secreted by the reproductive organs of aromatic plants, that is:

- *from the aerial parts (flowers, leaves, seeds, stems or branches)*
- *from the underground parts (roots or rhizome)*
- *From the whole plant or from a part of it (leaves, bark) it is extracted, usually by steam distillation in a still, the essence of the plant.*

The process of essential oil extraction allows to capture the most delicate and fragile components present in plants.

DIY essential oils: how to make them

You can, however, make your own essential oils with a distiller still. With this device you can, in fact, distil at home.

Without a still, you can use the maceration of plants in an oily base to obtain the oleolite or oil macerate.

Essential oil by steam distillation. You can extract the essential oils from the plants and make the hydrolate (distilled plant water) yourself by steam distillation with a device called a hydro-distiller or still.

Oleolite by maceration in vegetable oil. You can macerate herbs and flowers from your garden and vegetable garden in a basic vegetable oil (carrier oil). You will get concentrates that are less strong than those commercially available.

Distillation in brief

The process of steam distillation extracts and separates the volatile and aromatic oils from the plant material thanks to the steam, in fact, and to make it you need a still. This apparatus is preferably made of copper because of its better filtering capacity and it is made of few main elements:

- boiler, located at the bottom, where water is brought to boil in order to generate steam which, passing through the herbs, captures the oils
- filter column, with a grid, placed above the boiler, where the parts of the plant from which the oil is to be extracted are placed. Here is the passage of the current of steam generated by the boiler on plants and herbs.
- cooling pre-chamber, located in the upper part, where steam, now rich in volatile aromas, is collected and then conveyed to the condenser.
- cooling system, where the vapor condenses in order to return to a liquid state, usually a lateral coil around which passes cold water which is never in direct contact with the vapor. From here the water falls into a container and is arranged in an upper layer of essential oil and a lower layer of hydrolate, and it is collected from the tap.

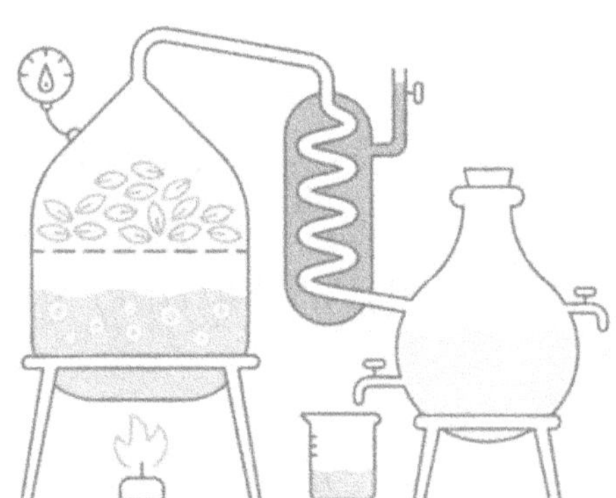

The distillation process is carried out as follows: the water vapor coming from the boiler, passes through the filter column containing the plants. The plant tissues break releasing the essential oil and aromatic molecules. The vapor is enriched by these substances and collects in the pre-chamber, here a nozzle and a small tube bring it to the cooling coil. The coil ends in a glass in which the oil-water solution is poured.

The result of the distillation is a mixture of flavored distilled water (hydrolate) and essential oil. The lighter, thicker oil separates from the watery part and is collected through a tap.

How to do essential oil distillation: the various steps

The distillation operation usually takes from 1 hour and a half to 3 hours. During the process it may be necessary to add cold water on the cooling coil or top up the water in the boiler.

1. Put mineral or distilled water in the boiler until it touches the filter column grid.
2. Place fresh or dried plants or flowers in the filter column over which steam will pass, thus loading it with essential oil molecules by distillation.
3. Close the lid of the boiler.
4. Light a camping stove underneath, or alternatively use the kitchen stove in distillers without iterative heating, or start the heating.
5. Open the cooling water tap when the boiler temperature is 50°. Steam, charged with essential oil, must condense by passing through a glass spiral cooled by cold water and then it is collected in a glass beaker provided with a tap.
6. Recover the distilled water or hydrolate, obtained from the condensation during the whole distillation process with the tap placed at the bottom of the glass.

7. Recover the oil that condenses at the same time as water but, being lighter, floats on top of water in the same glass, from the same faucet, taking care to remove the hydrolate first.

You can keep them in small 10-20 ml bottles of dark glass and in a dark and cool place, not over 20°. It is also good in the fridge. Use a few drops at a time to be taken with a pipette or dropper.

Diy Oleolite

You will have a vegetable oil as your base (carrier oil). You can use olive oil available in every kitchen for convenience, or more neutral skin-friendly oils like almond oil or wheat germ oil.

There are two main methods for preparing DIY oil macerates, the cold or hot method. Let's see them in detail.

DIY Oleolite: Cold Method

Let's start with the cold method:

- 250 ml vegetable oil
- 1 cup 250 ml of fresh leaves, herbs or flowers

Preparation. Put the leaves and flowers in a plastic bag, close it and crush it lightly, for example with a wooden pestle or rolling pin. This operation serves to cause the oil to come out from the aerial parts of the plant.

Immediately afterwards put them in a large glass jar with a wide mouth and a cork together with the vegetable oil to which the medicinal plants will gradually yield their aroma. Put it in a warm place, but not in direct contact with sun rays, for a period ranging from 24 to 48 hours. Then filter it with the help of a cotton gauze.

In order to strengthen the fragrance and concentration of the oil, get some fresh herbs and flowers in the same quantities (they should fit in a 250 ml cup) which you will put again in the closed plastic bag. Once crushed, add them to the oil in the previous container.

Again leave them to rest in the oil for another 24-48 hours, then filter again. Repeat the ritual for another time and, eventually, one more time, until the intensity of the scent is enough to please you.

At the end of the procedure filter again with a cotton gauze and with the help of a funnel transfer everything in a dark glass bottle provided with a dropper cap or in a normal bottle to be kept in a dark place.

Diy Oleolite: Hot Method

An alternative method to this is the hot method, that is you cook the oil and the herbs. In this case get yourself:

- 250 ml of vegetable oil
- 1/4 cup of 250 ml of fresh leaves, herbs or flowers

Preparation. Put the herbs intact (without crushing them as in the first procedure) in the oil and put everything to cook over low heat in a large, thick-bottomed saucepan in a bain-marie, for 6 hours. Let it cool down, filter with a cotton gauze and then transfer everything in a dark bottle for the use you are going to do.

The essential oil obtained in this way must be used within 6 months from its making, after every use it is necessary to remember to rinse hands and avoid touching eyes. Never dilute the oil with water.

Ointments and Salves

Ointments and salves have mainly a curative purpose and are very useful to always carry with you as first aid remedies. Let's learn how to make them by ourselves.

Basic recipe for 50 g of Ointment

Ingredients:

- 8 g of beeswax
- 40 ml of vegetable oil or oleolite
- 15 drops maximum of essential oils

Procedure:

Melt the wax together with the vegetable oil over very low heat. In the cooling phase add the essential oils. The properties of the ointment depend on the essences that we add.

Oleoliths are bought in herbalist shops and are derived from the maceration of the plant in oil instead of distillation with alcohol. Some medicinal plants such as arnica, helichrysum and marigold are not well suited for distillation and for this reason oleoliths are used. In the recipe they replace the basic vegetable oil or they complement it.

In the case of plants that lend themselves to distillation is very good to use essential oils. Once the ointment is obtained, pour it into white or brown glass jars. Stir from time to time with a small spoon until completely cooled to avoid the formation of a crust on the surface.

Healing Syrups

Herbs, roots and berries in particular, since ancient times, were preserved in curative and invigorating preparations, elixirs of long life, in which the most varied qualities of herbaceous families were secretly mixed.

Aloe Syrup

Ingredients:

- 150 g aloe pulp;
- 250 g of honey;
- 2 tablespoons of rum or grappa;

Before proceeding with the preparation, remember these rules:

1) All steps of the preparation, from the choice of the Aloe leaf, through the shake and up to the storage and consumption must be done ALL IN THE SHELF OF INTENSE LIGHT;

2) The chosen plant must not have been watered for at least 5/6 days.

Preparation:

Aloe leaf should be cut preferably in the evening or in the dark because light ruins its properties.

Clean the Aloe leaf with a dry cloth and remove the side thorns;

Blend the leaves initially with the intermittent button, taking care that the product does not overheat. It is therefore advisable to operate the blender intermittently;

When everything has been blended, add honey and blend, again intermittently, making sure there are no lumps;

Pour the product in a wide-necked dark-colored bottle and wrap it in aluminium foil (the neck and the cap of the bottle as well);

Keep in the fridge (vegetable compartment) until the end of the product (max. 15 days);

Take a spoonful of syrup, three times a day, 20 minutes before each meal;

The product must be consumed within 15 days.

Give the aloe vera the right amount of time to act, at least 3 to 4 months so that your body can adapt to the medicine;

Sage Syrup

Sage liqueur can be drunk immediately, as soon as it is bottled: the properties of sage, calming, soothing, women's friend par excellence (regularizes the menstrual cycle, helps in menopause to calm the sudden changes in body temperature), expectorant, hypoglycemic and also digestive, in very small quantities (1 teaspoon per day) as a restorative and invigorating, especially on cold winter days.

Ingredients:

- 60 sage leaves,
- 500 ml of brandy (neutral not the already flavored),
- 200 grams of semi-whole cane sugar.

Dust the sage leaves well from impurities and possible insects: put the leaves in a 700 ml container with a high neck. Fill the container with the brandy and seal it with an airtight stopper, the sage leaves that will not be covered with the brandy will oxidize and the liquor will take on a typical brownish color. Shake well the container and leave it in infusion for 30 days on a sunny windowsill, in case you prepare it in winter or autumn make sure it is placed on a balcony where the sun shines more. After 30 days the recipe is completed with the preparation of the syrup: simmer sugar in 200 ml of water until it is completely dissolved, then let it cool. Strain the sage infusion through a strainer into a large bowl, then add the syrup and mix well with a wooden spoon (do not use metal). Bottle in sterilized bottles (20 minutes from boiling in a pot full of water) and decorate with one or two sage leaves soaked in brandy. It will keep for 12 months.

Rose Hip Berry Syrup

This syrup is taken in case of sore throat and cough, the recommended dose is 3-4 tablespoons per day, away from meals.

Ingredients for one litre of syrup:

- half a litre of water,
- 500 gr of honey,
- 100 grams of rosehip berries,
- 10-15 grams of mint leaves,
- 10 ml of propolis tincture.

Remove the seeds from the rosehips and the internal hairs, leaving only the pulp; with the help of a pestle, puree them. Bring a pot of water to a boil and, as soon as it comes to a boil, pour in the rose berry puree, lower the heat and cook for at least 30 minutes. Turn off the heat and add the mint, keeping it in infusion for at least 10 minutes with the pan covered in order not to evaporate the active ingredients. With the help of a strainer on which you will have placed a gauze, filtered the drink and squeezed the gauze itself. To the liquid add 500 grams of honey: if the honey does not melt, put the herbal tea back on the fire without boiling it, until the honey melts, then let it cool, add the propolis and stir quickly to prevent the propolis from sticking to the pot. Bottle this syrup in a sterilized dark glass container. It will keep in the refrigerator for up to six months.

Cinnamon Syrup

Ingredients:

- 5 grams cinnamon rind,
- 10 grams of gentian,
- 20 juniper berries,
- 5 grams of mint,
- 10 grams of lemon peel (yellow part only),
- 1,5 grams of vanilla in stick,
- 320 grams of 95° alcohol,
- 250 grams of water,
- 500 grams of sugar.

Crush vanilla and cinnamon in a mortar and let them macerate in alcohol in a hermetically sealed glass jar for about 10 days shaking it twice a day. Filter and squeeze the herbs well then add the sugar with which you will have made a syrup by dissolving it as usual in water heated over low heat.

Amalgamating everything, let it rest for one day, refilter and bottle it closing with wax, consume it after 3 months. This elixir, which you will be able to give to your guests without disfiguring them, will be drunk before or after meals in the quantity of half a glass. Cinnamon has excellent tonic and stimulating properties therefore it is an active stomach stimulator.

Licorice Syrup

Ingredients

- 300 ml of water
- 200 g of cane sugar

- *60 g of pure licorice*

Combine the pure licorice in a powerful blender and mix until an impalpable powder is obtained.

Pour the water into a small saucepan and bring to the boil. Pour in the whole cane sugar and stir until completely dissolved. Then add the pure licorice powder and continue to stir for 2-3 minutes, taking care not to let the liquid spill out of the pot.

If necessary strain the syrup through a sieve.

Pour the licorice syrup into small bottles or glass jars with screw caps and refrigerate for 2 months.

Mint Syrup

Ingredients:

- 50 grams peppermint,
- 200 grams of 95° alcohol,
- ¼ litre dry white wine,
- 2 lemon peels (only the yellow part).

Soak the mint leaves in a jar together with the alcohol for about two days, then add the wine and the lemon peels, let it rest for another two days and filter. Consume fresh in the doses of 1-3 glasses a day. Mint liquor, besides being an excellent thirst quencher, is also a stimulant for the nervous system. You can vary the recipe by adding 150 grams of honey: the liqueur will gain in flavor making it even more pleasing to the palate.

Elderberry Syrup

Elderberry syrup is a sweet beverage not to be confused with elderberry juice (which is obtained from fruits/berries) or with elderberry grappa (alcohol based).

In herbal medicine are used elder flowers and leaves (Sambucus nigra L.), but to make the syrup we will use only flowers which have properties:

- diuretic,
- diaphoretic (that is it increases sweating favouring the elimination of toxins. Moreover, it lowers the body temperature by fighting fever).

Preparation time: 10 minutes + 24 hours of rest

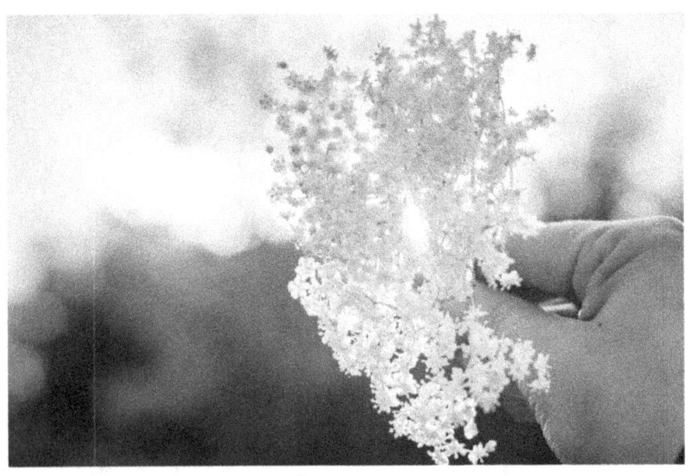

Ingredients:

- 2 Lt water
- 2 Kg of sugar
- 2 limes or organic lemons
- 15 tufts of elder flowers (picked from a plant that is far from the pollution of the streets)
- 50 g of citric acid (available in pharmacies. To make this syrup without citric acid, increase the amount of lime/lemon to 4)

Procedure:

In a large pot we put all the elderflowers without washing them (you can whisk them a bit to get any insects out). It is very important not to wash the flowers in order not to lose the aroma.

Next, we pour the sugar, water and citric acid over our flowers. We stir a bit to allow the sugar to dissolve more easily and pour in the limes / lemons simply cut in half or in rounds (without squeezing them).

At this point we cover everything with cling film and leave it to macerate cold for about 24 hours stirring every now and then with a wooden spoon (about every 2-3 hours) in order to facilitate the complete dissolution of sugar.

After 24 hours the lime/lemon are removed (they can be squeezed for other preparations) and the syrup is filtered with a strainer. Completely filtered, a clear and yellow syrup is obtained.

The elderflower syrup is ready! You can proceed, then, to bottling and store in the refrigerator for about 1 month - 1 month and a half.

Ginger Syrup

Ingredients:

- 180g brown sugar
- 60g ginger root
- 400g water
- a teaspoon of lemon juice

Peel and chop the ginger, place it in a saucepan with the water and sugar.

Cook over high heat until it comes to a boil, then lower the heat and continue cooking for an hour.

After this time, filter the mixture through a sieve and add a teaspoon of lemon juice to the syrup. Stir well. *A little tip, the discarded pieces of ginger can be dried and then pulverized with the mixer and so ginger powder for everyone and nothing is wasted!

Pour into previously sterilized glass bottles and cap.

The ginger syrup can be stored in a cool place in the pantry and kept away from light. Once opened store in the refrigerator and consume within a few days to ensure freshness. I suggest for this reason to use rather small bottles in order to use it in the shortest time possible.

A small deposit on the bottom will be completely normal as the color is not transparent but still golden!

Holy Pipe

There is no doubt that the Pipe is the sacred object par excellence for most Native American tribes. The Pipe gave, in fact, meaning, importance and order to rituals that celebrated life.

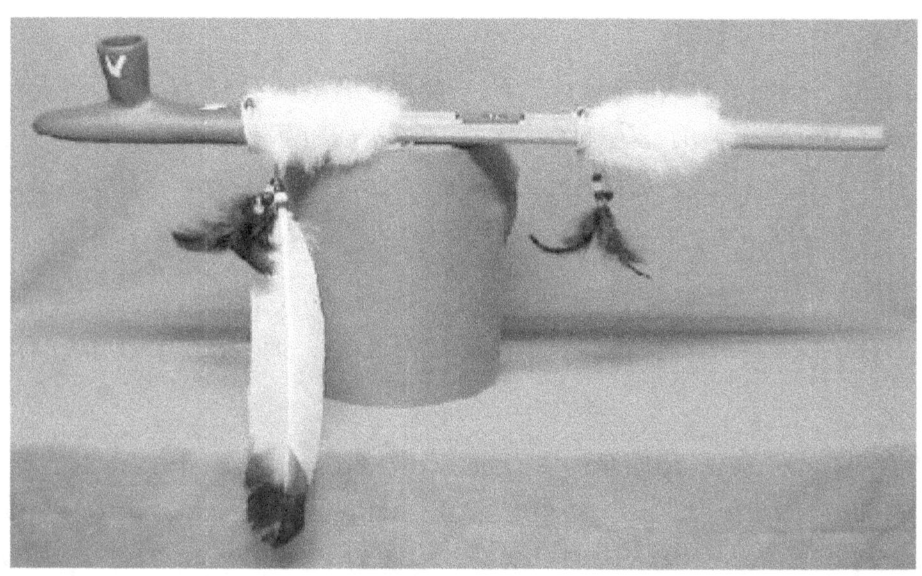

The best known is surely the T-shaped Pipe, also called "Calumet", smoked when a peace treaty was stipulated, so much so that it became famous among the whites as the "Pipe of Peace", even if this term could be reductive, not rendering entirely the profound meaning of the Pipe, not a simple object, according to the spirituality of the Natives, but a "living thing", dwelling of the power of the Great Spirit.

Ritual Pipes were, and are kept, when not in use, in sacred wrappings of decorated buckskin or deer skin, and the two parts are kept separate because being endowed with great power, the act of keeping them connected would be considered sacrilegious.

The Sacred Pipe has always played a key role in the Creation Stories that describe and explain the origins of many tribes. The pipe is an integral part of the ceremony, it is present whenever there is an important decision to be made, from making peace to declaring war, when there is a need to ensure a good hunt or encourage good work, in healing practices. The pipe symbolizes the perfect balance, the union between Heaven and Earth, male and female, spiritual world and physical world; even the name, Chanumpa, according to the Lakota diction, is the union between Cha, wood, and Numpa.

It is in fact made up of two parts: the stove, ihupa, is the Tree of Life, and is made of maple wood, and the stove, pahu, in the shape of a T or L, which represents the world, the creation. In fact, all Pipe stoves of all North American tribes are made from a red stone called Inyan sha, pipestone in English.

It is the "Catlinite", found in only one place in the world, in Pipestone, Minnesota.

It is thought that excavation work in this area began around the seventeenth century and the large stone blocks or pipe stoves already worked were transported across the continent by Plains tribes to areas such as the Pecos and New Mexico, where they traded with tribes in the Southwest.

The ritual of the Sacred Pipe and the Sacred Pipe itself have a value for the Natives that goes beyond what many people believe, a value that is above all Spiritual; in fact the Sacred Pipe is smoked in many other rites and celebrations.

Seven Laws of the Holy Pipe

"Seven are the Sacred Laws that govern the life of the Lakota People, which were given to us, along with the Sacred Pipe by the White Buffalo Woman.

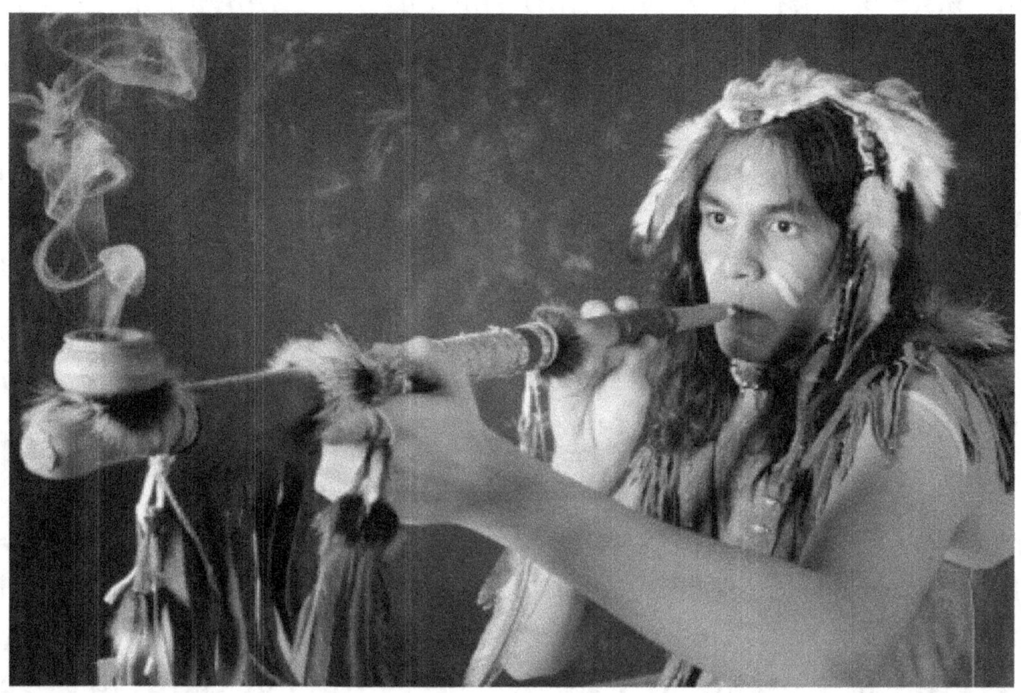

Seven are the Sacred Ceremonies we were taught, so that we could live in harmony with the universe. Seven are the Stars of the Big Dipper, representing the progenitors of the groups that constitute the Council of the Seven Fires and seven are the subdivisions of the Tetonwan, "those who live in the prairie".

Seven are the sacred places located in Cante Wamakognake, the "Heart of all that exists", the Paha Sapa, the Black Hills. To each of these sacred places correspond the Seven Sacred Constellations of the Sky.

Finally, seven are the Pleiades Stars, the place where the Lakota lived when they still belonged to the World of the Spirit.

One of the most beautiful stories that the Lakota children heard from their grandparents, during the cold winter evenings, sitting around the fire, was that of the White Buffalo Woman.

It tells of how, many generations ago, the Lakota people lived in great difficulty. They were hungry, they quarrelled, the brothers fought among themselves. Even the winters seemed colder and harder to overcome.

It was in one of those cold seasons that two hunters left the camp in search of bison to hunt. For days and days, they searched for tracks, but to no avail. When disappointed, they decided to return to the camp, they noticed a solitary figure approaching from the west.

This figure had a strange gait; not the normal human way of walking, but a strange floating, which convinced the two hunters that it must be a sacred entity. When it came within a short distance of the two Lakota, they realized it was a beautiful woman, wearing a white buckskin dress superbly embroidered with porcupine quills, in brilliant colors.

She wore long, black, shiny hair, loose on her shoulders, except for a braid, on her left side, wrapped with buffalo skin. In her hands she held a fan made of sprigs of sage and she wore an envelope made of leather hanging from her back.

Her superb beauty aroused in one of the two hunters the desire to possess her, while the other, with reverential fear, paid her the respect due to a sacred being.

The Woman, turning to the first hunter, said that, if she really wanted, she could have what she so desired, but for this her life would have been consumed in a very short time.

In fact, in a few moments, the man's body dissolved, filled with worms and leaving only a pile of dried up bones.

The other hunter, terrified by what had happened to his companion, was calmed down by the woman, who, in a sweet tone, told him to go back to his people, to gather the elders, the chiefs and the spiritual interpreters in a large circle, in the middle of which they would have to erect a large tipi.

The next day, the Woman would have visited the People, bringing as a gift an object and some teachings, which had the purpose of reminding forever the Lakota people of the sacredness of life.

This is what happened. The next morning, once the Woman entered the field circle, she entered the tipi and sat at the place of honour, where sage had been sprinkled.

First, from the burden she carried on her back she pulled out a large pipe with a wooden blowpipe and a red stone stove, adorned with mottled eagle feathers. He explained to them that the stove, carved from stone, represented the earth and the blood of the people, while the pipe, carved from wood, symbolized all the beings living on earth.

The eagle feathers, as well as the symbol of the People of the Winged, represented the message of Tunkasila.

He showed them how they should use the pipe, during prayers, offering it first to the Four Directions, then to Heaven and then to Mother Earth.

He explained how the smoke coming out of the pipe would carry their prayers and voices up to heaven.

After that he told the Lakota about the Seven Sacred Ceremonies that would be the center of their religion from then on and showed how to celebrate them. Then he spoke of how each individual was to fulfill his duty first within the family, then within the nation.

For this purpose the Seven Sacred Laws were given, saying that only the strict observance of these rules would allow the Lakota people to live a harmonious and balanced life. When he had finished, he stepped out of his tipi, making a turn according to the path of the sun, and headed for the edge of the camp circle.

He turned one last time to look at his people and as soon as he had passed the edge of the field, he turned into a black male bison. He began to gallop in the same direction from which he had come, then changed the color of his coat, first brown, then red, and then finally turned into a white bison that disappeared into the horizon.

That was the first and last time anyone saw her, and no one heard from her again.

The concepts expressed by the Seven Sacred Laws that the Sacred Woman gave to the Lakota People are profound but also simple.

1. The first Law is Wacante Ognake, which means "To carry in the Heart the good of the People." It is therefore an invitation to generosity. We do not own the land, but we belong to the land. We

are its custodians. And the same thing applies to all forms of life that populate it.

2. The second Law, very important, must almost become a second skin for the Lakota. Wawoyuonihan, "Respect and love all the creatures that surround us", whether they be of the Two-Legged People, the Four-Legged People, the Winged People, the Fish People, the Vegetable People or the Mineral People. The meaning of Wacin Tanka is "To have a great mind."

3. This is the third law that reminds the Lakota to be patient and tolerant.

4. The Fourth Law, Wowahunsila, teaches to have mercy and compassion toward all creatures, as well as to love and respect them.

5. The defining word of the Fifth Law is an invitation to modesty and humility: Wowahwala. Those who wish to possess humility and modesty must be silent and quiet. In the middle of the word, we find the sound "hwa," which means "to fall asleep." In fact, sleep is also a further search for understanding. And it is also through dreams and visions that we must try to understand what is happening around us.

6. The Sixth Law is Woohitike and reminds us that we must be bold, courageous and fearless. We must not be afraid to live by our principles.

7. The last and seventh law is Woksape...the pursuit of wisdom. We will only achieve this state if we have managed to live by the first six laws. In order to remind ourselves of the importance that these rules contain, every night we must raise our eyes to the sky and look at the place from which we came: the Pleiades.

And to never forget the importance of living a good life, we look at the Sacred Pipe and look at the woman, whom we consider sacred.

The Seven Sacred Ceremonies that the White Bison Woman taught us, explaining that these were seven different ways that the Lakota would have from then on, to send voices to Tunkasila, still represent today, the essence of the Lakota religion.

Lakota Rituals

1- RITE - Onikare or also: INIPI: it is the sacred rite of purification, the sweat lodge is sacred, it represents the universe, and in it everything is contained, the incandescent stones in the center of the hut sprinkled with fresh water produce purifying steam, one prays for the people, for their loved ones, for themselves, one purifies from earthly negativity, at the end of the rite one is "reborn" with a new soul and ready to face daily difficulties again. Sacred herbs such as sage, sweet grass, cedar, juniper are used during the ceremony is burned on hot stones and "rubbed" on the body of each participant.

2- ISNATI-AWICALOWAN RITE: it is the rite of "female puberty": the ceremony - reserved to young women - celebrates the sacred passage from adolescence to adulthood, the young women receive instructions not only from their mother, aunts and grandmothers, but also from the "sacred woman", who has the task of guiding and leading the young girls. The rite is also the vehicle through which a "spiritual bond" is created with Wope, that is "the white bison woman". All this takes place in a particular "tepee" (the traditional cone-shaped tent of the nomadic peoples of the great plains), specially prepared to celebrate the ceremony.

3- RITE HAMBLECHEYAPI: that is "to lament for having a vision, can also be translated as: crying for the vision". The rite is carried out by young people guided by an intercessor of the sacred, is performed to obtain a vision, to clarify the meaning of a dream, to seek advice from *higher forces in difficult times or when you have to pass from youth to adulthood, you choose a sacred hill where the subject, always under the careful guidance of the Spiritual mediator, remains for 4 days without water and without food, without clothes, only with his sacred pipe and a fur of bison, at the end of 4 days will immediately follow a ritual inipi and then after smoking the sacred pipe, the spiritual leader, will help the subject to interpret and clarify the vision had.*

4- *RITE HUNKAYAPI: is the ceremony of union with ties of kinship: with it is celebrated the entry into the family in the extended sense that is called "TIOSPAYE" of a new individual. During the ceremony, are given to the new family member precise indications of his duties towards the new members of his family, there is a man who leads the ceremony using, the sacred pipe, a horse hair, an eagle feather, and "incensing" the participants with sacred sage, before the conclusion the new member and the head of the family must express their consent, before all, on the new mutual duties accepted and declare to accept each other.*

5- *RITE WIWANYAG WACHIPI: it is the rite of the sacred dance of the sun, in the thought and "philosophy" of the natives, everything has a spherical, circular aspect: everything moves following the "natural movement of the sun and with it that of the earth and the stars". Also the place where the Dance of the Sun takes place is circular, built with wooden poles in order to form a perfect circle. Exactly in the center of the circle a big hole is dug, representing our mother, the earth. Inside this hole the "Wakachan" will be placed, that is the sacred poplar tree that represents the male element, the antenna that will send to the universe and to the "Great Father" our sufferings and our supplications. Each dancer ties his "rope" to the high branches of the poplar tree, which represents the umbilical cord that once tied us to our mother. The incisions that the spiritual leader makes on each dancer, exactly at the level of the pectoral muscles, cutting from one side to the other the flesh and sliding two splinters either in bone or in wood, cause the physical pain, accentuated by the rope that is fixed to these splinters. Each dancer with tension movements will try to tear his flesh, freeing himself from the rope and from the splinters with enormous physical pain. Such suffering is similar to that which our mother felt one day in order to give us the greatest gift: LIFE. In this way the dancers give back to their mother, the earth, part of these sufferings and of their blood, to thank first of all for the life they had and for all that with it has been and will be given to us, moreover the rite intends to express the humility that every dancer shows by giving in sacrifice what is most precious: his physical body and his blood, remaking in a symbolic way what was done at the beginning of creation. Inside the circle and for 4 days without eating or drinking. We dance praying and sacrificing for others, for the suffering of our loved ones, for a better world. This rite, which takes different procedural forms depending on the tribe that practices it, always has a common meaning that is described. The Lakota thought that, suffering at the center of the sacred circle, they assumed on themselves all the sufferings of their people and that their sacrificed body, represented the ignorance of man. Therefore, with these ceremonies, they tried to be as humble as possible and to free themselves from any lower "negativity", all for the good of their People. The dance of the sun was held, and still takes place today, in the summer months when the moon was full, and the camp was filled with joy and at the same time of deep sacredness. Warriors and women, wore their best clothes and sometimes different clans would gather together to celebrate this important event.*

6- *RITE TAPA WANKA YAP, is the ritual of "throwing the ball or sphere": in this ceremony is used a ball made with a bison skin, inside which are inserted hairs of bison itself, a young girl, is placed in the middle of the sacred field and rows of people are arranged to the 4* cardinal points: west-north-east-south. The girl throws the ball in turn in each of the 4 directions always starting from west, and each person in the group grabs the ball offering it to the 4 quadrants of the universe and then towards the "zenith" and then throw it back to the girl in the center. We can say that the ball represents the strength of the "great spirit" and the 4 teams of people the entities of the 4 quadrants of the universe and the world and that grabbing the ball, so what it represents, that is the "great spirit", they grab with it also the knowledge.

7- RITE WANAGI YUHA: it is the rite of the custody of the soul, this rite has risked to disappear almost totally because of the governmental and Christian impositions against the spirituality of the Natives, fortunately, like the other rituals it has survived and today, in some reserves it is practiced. When a family member dies his or her spirit is kept for a period that can last from 6 to 12 months. The spirit is kept by the relatives, until with an appropriate ritual is returned to its origin; the relatives of the deceased offer most of their belongings to the needy, in memory of the dead. A lock of hair is cut, by the intercessor of the Sacred One, from the front of the head of the deceased and then wrapped in leather or cloth, it is kept in a sacred manner for 4 days. After a period, that as said can vary from 6 months to 12 months, in a special Tepee, built for the occasion, the spiritual mediator, performs a particularly complex ceremony, of course using the sacred pipe: he takes from the relatives of the deceased the bundle with the hair and releases outside the spirit of "the one who is no longer with us". The time of tears ends and the relatives will then remember the deceased with joy, as he is now in a place far from human misfortune and suffering of life.

There are other rituals, still practiced on the Rosebud, Pine Ridge and Cheyenne River reservations, such as the Ywuipi ritual, which is a very powerful healing ritual with which the intercessor of the sacred, calls animal spirits, and human beings now passed into the spiritual world, to help those present at the ritual in physical and spiritual healing. It is a nightly ritual that began with the spiritual intercessor known as Horn Chips "Wopthua", circa 1840.

Sacred pipe ritual

The tobacco used was often mixed with the inner bark of the willow creating a fragrant mixture called: "Kinnikinnik" and among the Lakota "cansasa".

This mixture did not have, due to the small amount of tobacco, the harmful properties of today's tobacco. The smoke of the tobacco brought up the prayers offered up to reach the "great father" so that they were answered. There were many occasions when the sacred pipe was smoked: to celebrate an event, to honour a guest, to ward off negative events that could affect the family or the field, or for a relative who was dying, for an abundant hunt, for a birth, for peace, etc.:

The wooden blowpipe was joined with the stove and then here is that the sacred pipe, could express all its power: in the same way in which a man and a woman are united, giving rise to the life of a new being, so the union of the two elements of the pipe, create a powerful "antenna" transmission of prayer to the great Creator. To Him come the prayers represented by the tobacco potholders that are offered and deposited inside the stove itself. Before being inserted into the pipe, each tobacco pot is sprinkled with the smoke of sacred sage. When the whole stove has been filled with tobacco, it is first offered to the four quadrants of the universe (always starting from west to east), then to heaven and earth, and then smoked. Once the pipe has been offered to a *person, this person must always be sincere and his words must never be able to "hurt the heart" of those present, because the truth must always be told.*

Once the smoking is finished, the ashes in the stove will be thrown into the fire or placed on a sacred altar (usually a flat stone on which sacred herbs are burned) and the two parts of the pipe divided and placed wrapped in a skin or a cloth. No woman who is in her menstrual cycle can approach or touch the sacred pipe, because in this period the woman is particularly sacred because she is purifying herself, therefore the strength of her sacredness would affect the energy of the sacred pipe.

Every owner adorned his pipe in a different way according to the visions he had, or to the instructions of certain "men of medicine" who could suggest to use certain colors or certain decorations, each of which had a precise meaning not only aesthetic but also practical.

For example, using parts of the eagle was meant to represent the strength of the sun and the "great spirit".

Yana Nashua

BOOK 3

Native American Nations

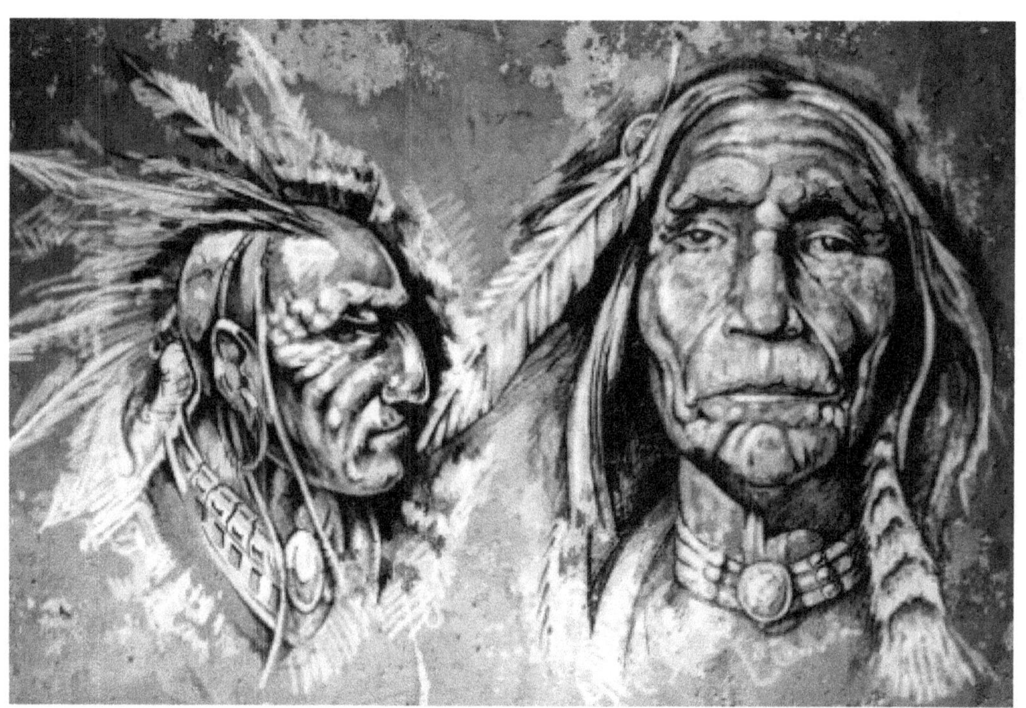

Yana Nashua

Natural Peoples and the Relationship with Animals

Although the planet seems to be pervaded by a rampant mentality that allows any abomination on other species, in reality there are cultures based on principles of respect for the planet and for all forms of life.

We have been accustomed for a long time to see how the intimate relationship between man and the mystery that animates existence and gives meaning to human presence itself passes through the various forms of religions that have been present for centuries on the planet. However, there are other cultures that do not depend on the religious beliefs introduced by the various prophets and their specific revelations. We refer to Natural Peoples, cultures that have related to existence without intermediaries, allowing each individual to freely refer to the mystery that gives life and meaning to existence. These peoples have been fought for centuries by the great historical religions, they have been subjected to violence of all kinds and have been deprived of their spiritual dignity to be forcibly converted in order to deny their experiential reality. Today, Natural Peoples are being rediscovered by History and are making people talk about them.

Natural Peoples, because of their emblematic character, represent a historical case. They are also often referred to as indigenous peoples, tribal peoples or native peoples of the planet. Natural Peoples are those cultures that do not have an ethical and spiritual reference in the great religions that have appeared in history and in the cultures that originated from them. These peoples live and propose their own specific way of living and relating to life.

Ultimately, the concept of natural peoples includes all those ethnic groups that have developed a spiritual culture outside the context of the great historical religions. As an example, we can cite the cultures of the Native Americans, the Indians of Central and South America, the Australian Aborigines, the natives of Oceania, the African and Asian Natives, as well as the Celtic populations of northern Europe. In practice, they are the natives of all continents, those cultures existing on the entire planet that maintain intact their relationship with Nature without dogmatic-religious intermediaries.

Natural Peoples base their sociality on a natural principle of peaceful aggregation of individuals, thus creating a synergy that is the result of a common goal of individuals: individual survival through the strength of the collective contribution.

The social forms of Natural Peoples have a natural continuity and are transmitted over time for a spontaneous use of social aggregation, not contemplating concepts such as nationalism, but on the contrary opening up to the universality offered by the planet and the universe beyond it.

The love that Natural Peoples have for the planet makes them feel part of the universe and of the Earth as the environmental dimension in which individuals were born and grew up. An experience of love and respect for Mother Earth, which she deserves as an emanation of the mystery that gave birth to everything.

Basing their life experience on these philosophical assumptions, Natural Peoples consequently conceive of society as a natural support for the needs *and experience of the individual. A synergistic tool that distributes its potential according to individual needs and with the collective contribution to the maintenance of that tool.*

On the basis of this philosophical vision, Natural Peoples do not conceive of their society as an elitist factor of man, an identity closed in on itself, but rather as an instrument that opens its use, according to specific possibilities, towards a participation in the environment together with all the other forms of life on the planet.

Natural Peoples integrate the environment in which their society develops, according to their own needs, but maintaining respect for nature in all its manifestations, without altering the specific rhythms of the place of settlement, but adapting to them in order to derive greater well-being from the resources offered naturally and without ruining any ecosystem that ultimately produces environmental disorder and turns against their own society.

Yana Nashua

The Relationship with the Environment in its Global meaning

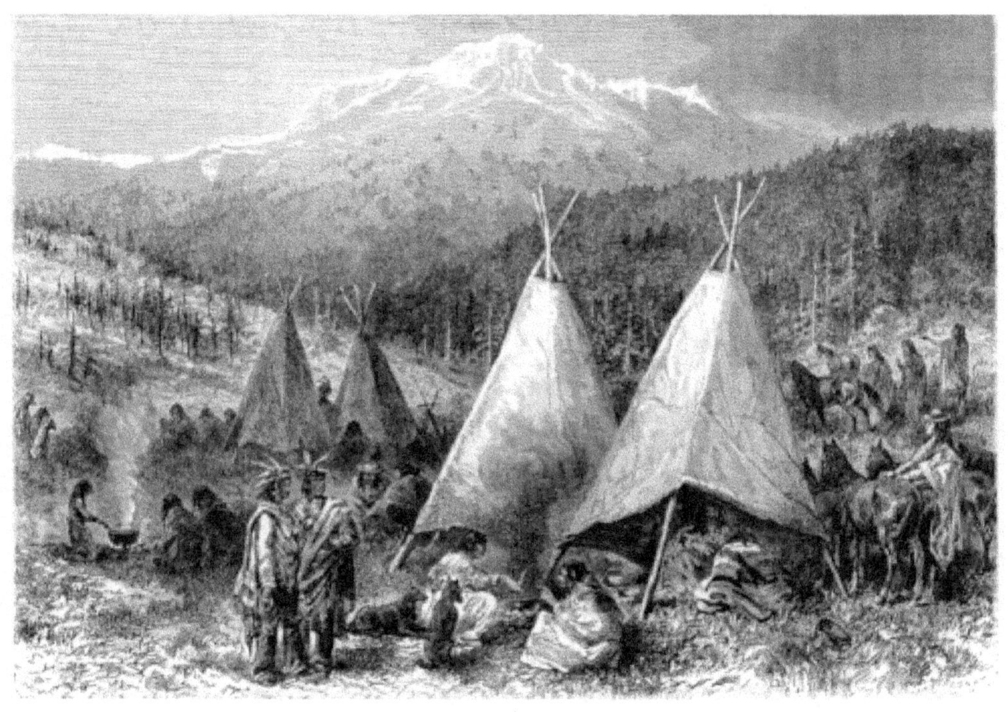

Natural Peoples express respect for life and nature by living in the perspective of the reality of the Mystery that animates the universe and that unites everyone in the same experience and existential substance.

These peoples live in the conception of a universe of which man is an integral part, an experiential quality in transit, engaged in a process of transmutation that does not necessarily exclude other forms of life. A process that affects all of existence and that has manifested itself in this corner of the universe as well.

For natural peoples, the Earth is seen as an ecosystem in which man appeared alongside other species, and from which man himself draws the experience of his evolution towards the Mystery, that great Mystery from which he was drawn at the moment of his birth. The Earth is poetically seen as an entity, mother of all life forms on the planet, in the conception of belonging to a single planetary family that includes all living creatures.

From this concept comes the need for a harmonious relationship, solidarity and reciprocity with the environment. Each individual is thus to interact with the environment and individual needs arise from participatory attitudes within the ecosystem.

The universalistic vision of natural peoples leads to the birth of respect and love for life in all its forms, leads to give equal dignity to every race and every species, the recognition of consciousness and feelings to animals, solidarity and equality between all living forms of the Earth and, eventually, of the cosmos.

Respect for the environment is born as an integral part of an ecosystem to which man also belongs, who cannot draw resources for his own benefit and at the expense of other living forms and environmental balance, with the risk of being rejected or end up being in an impoverished and hostile environment.

The need to avoid wasting resources and damaging the environment arises in the name of future generations, as they also belong to a globality that goes beyond the concept of space and time. It highlights the respect for the environment seen as existence lived in its most sacred aspect, as a manifestation of the immanence of the Mystery.

Here we find again the concept and the symbolism of Mother Earth, dear to the natural peoples of the whole planet, as a metaphysical reference: the Mystery that materializes in a state of manifest existence and in a source of well-being and of energetic and therapeutic resources.

Nature, understood as a state of existence and as an intermediary with the Mystery, even becomes an inner mystical reference. To understand this concept we must refer to the symbolism of the dark cave: a cave with a single source of light represented by the sun rays that illuminate a portion and indicate the exit, where all men and other species live and in which all are equal and with the same potential, made different only by the perception of the Mystery that welds them to the nature of reality illuminated by the sun to go towards.

This is what, according to the Natural Peoples, can unite men and animals in a common spirituality, perfectly sharable, that brings them together and makes them participants in harmony and perhaps in the meaning of existence.

The Animal Question

Natural Peoples consider other forms of life as co-inhabitants of the same environment, not separated from humans because of the difference in forms, and with faculties almost equal to human ones.

The same thing does not happen in the majority society where, for specific reasons of religious origin, the other living forms are downgraded to simple functionalities present in nature and at the complete disposal of man for his every whim or use.

The planet is rich in manifestations of life other than that of man. Life that populates the air, the seas and the same lands on which humanity lives. The interaction of the majority society with other forms of life occurs mainly with what are commonly identified as animals.

They are stripped of every possible attribute of intelligence and feeling. So much so that the men of the majority society use them as ordinary food, a source of protein for their sustenance, favoured by a few commercial elites who thrive on the backs of these unsuspecting living beings. In this perspective, breeding and slaughter camps are opened and structured in an efficient and productive way.

The majority society is not limited only to the systematic slaughter of the animals in charge, but also uses them as slaves in areas where energy sources are limited and in the hands of specific and exclusive centres of power. In this case we are witnessing what was already happening among humans themselves in the productive societies of the past where, instead of a possible technological development, human slaves were used to perform the work. In the same way, the use of weak social classes by other minority classes able to exert their power over others began later.

In other cases, the killing of animals also occurs for the various orientations that are proper to the majority and productive society, as in the case of ritual killing practiced by religions or killing elevated to sport for the psychological needs of the class of hunters.

The majority society, however, pays for its violence with the disastrous results of the carnivorous diet on individuals and with the conflict that arises within the society itself.

The affirmation of the superiority of men over animals has led to the creation of categories, giving rise to a dangerous and deleterious principle that has resulted in the removal of man from harmony with nature. Principle that extended to humanity itself by creating racial and sexist supremacies. This deviation has generated unnecessary conflict and suffering and has slowed the progress of all humanity, leading it to deprive itself of the experience of other portions of the sky.

But this view of animals does not arise by chance, nor does it represent a factual situation. The problem arises from a precise vision of things that affects the attitude of men in their relationship with life and leads to accept truths acquired and not experienced.

A vision that conditions man in his daily choices and mortgages even science, which for its part does not base its thesis on a position of equidistance towards the problem of animals, but on religious positions that lead to study other species to understand whether or not they are able to express their own intelligence.

This view justifies that animals are seen as automata, that they can be enslaved and killed to be eaten or ritually sacrificed, and that this barbarity is even considered normal.

It is mistakenly thought that all native peoples are carnivores and hunters, and this may seem to contradict the respect that these peoples give to other species. In reality this is not the case. Those peoples who have been most consistent with their traditions do not eat animals. We have many examples: the ancient Hunza people of the Himalayas, a population known for its longevity, among which there is a notable presence of ultra-centenarians with a life expectancy that would be around 130 years. Or the Vilcabamba people of Ecuador, also with a life expectancy of around 130 years. Their diet is based on cereals and fruit grown by themselves without the use of chemicals. There are also the Guarani of South America, essentially frugivorous, the natives of Mount Hagen in New Guinea who feed on raw vegetable foods, the Abkhazians of Georgia and many others. As for Native Americans, there is a stereotype of the Indian buffalo hunter, dressed in decorated skins, elaborate feathered headdresses and leather moccasins, housed in a leather tent, master of dogs and horses and uninterested in vegetables. But this lifestyle spread only a few centuries ago and does not correspond to most Native Americans of today or yesterday. In fact, the bison-related lifestyle is a direct result of European influence. In the diet of the Choctaw Indians of Mississippi and Oklahoma, the main dishes were vegetarian. An eighteenth-century French manuscript describes the vegetarian propensities of the Choctaw in building and eating. Dwellings were built not with hides, but with wood, mud, bark, and reeds. The main food, eaten daily in earthenware bowls, was a vegetarian soup made from corn, pumpkin and beans. Bread was made with maize and acorns.

Other typical dishes were roasted corn and a corn porridge. The ancient Choctaw were, first and foremost, farmers. Even clothes were made from vegetables, dresses with artistic embroidery for women and cotton pants for men. Also as for the Australian Aborigines, the testimonies of the tribes still existing today tell that their elders lived on a diet based on vegetable foods, such as nuts, seeds, fruits and vegetables, and that even today they find in the Australian bush all the nutrients and proteins necessary for their sustenance.

Animal Spirituality

The natural peoples of any continent, despite the geographical distance and the differences in culture and language, have in common a fundamental principle: spirituality based on contact with Nature. A Nature seen not only in its ecological aspect but above all as the depository of a great cosmic mystery. This concept leads them to see spirituality in every manifestation of the universe and in every form of life. Therefore respect for life is of utmost importance for these cultures.

According to the ancient traditions of the Natives of all continents, animals are not what they seem. Beyond their appearance they keep secrets related to the relationship with the invisible dimension of the transcendent. Each animal can be a spirit-guide for those who approach it, able to lead him beyond the door of the visible. These creatures are the totemic animals that the ancient traditions of the Natives of all continents, from Native Americans to the Celts, from Australian Aborigines to African Natives, going back to ancient Druidic shamanism, have identified as archetypal symbols that can open our horizons and arouse metaphysical insights. Very wise beings from whom we can receive profound teachings, because they have a natural and direct relationship with Mother Earth, and from whom we can learn to live in harmony with Nature and with ourselves.

According to ancient shamanic traditions, each of us has a totemic animal, or even more than one, depending on the periods of our lives or situations. They are not necessarily physical entities. They may manifest in a dream, or in a vision, or we may encounter them in a forest or in an everyday situation in a seemingly casual way. Sometimes they are closer to us than we think. Discreet and silent companions who accompany our lives as protectors who are always there when needed, even if we do not realize it.

This conception of animals, seen as guardians of a door to the Invisible, also makes us reflect on the meaning of their spirituality.

If existence manifests the property of a transmutation of its experiential quality, why attribute this property exclusively to humans?

Preconception relegates animals to the rank of automata without feelings, and this authorizes us to use them as objects. But observation without preconceptions relates humans to animals and allows us to discover an experience that is common to all forms of life.

Beyond prejudices on the subject, interesting and shocking discoveries can be made: one can discover that animals have feelings, that like man they feel a value of conscious suffering. One can discover that so-called "animals" are beings endowed with a self-awareness and consciously manage their lives in relation to the same existential questions that human beings ask themselves.

This discourse leads far, because it leads to realize that we cannot exclude a priori the possibility that, as happens among humans, even among animals may exist individuals capable of developing their own spirituality.

It is inevitable to wonder about the meaning of spirituality, extended to other species. It is inevitable to feel a sense of brotherhood that extends also to animals and that can unite us to the whole of existence.

Yana Nashua

The importance of animals for Native Americans

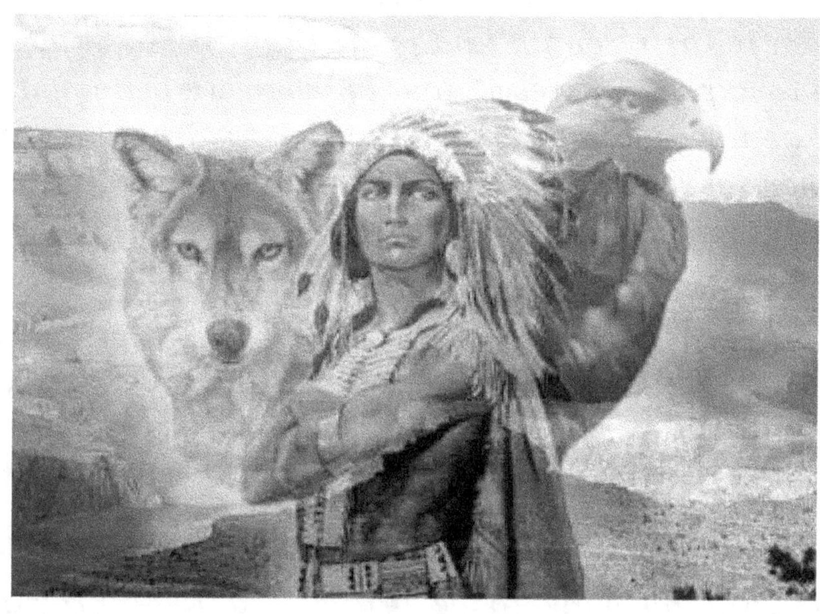

Animals have been a vital part of Plains Indians' lives. Most stories involve animals and other living things, when elders talk to children to the point of explaining the important qualities of each living thing.

Not only did the various animals and birds and other creatures provide food, shelter and other necessities, they taught lessons to many people and showed them how to create useful items as you will see from the story below.

Native Americans thank both the Creator and the spirit of the animal kill for food and hides, because they are linked to it in that the Creator created all living things for a purpose.

Animal Totems

Moose

Respect and esteem for one's being as well as recognizing that a creative process has been rightly completed, are qualities that well symbolize the moose in addition to the strength and pride that are highly developed. From it we can learn to express ourselves loudly when we feel joy at a feat or task completed, just as the moose in heat lets out its rallying cry in spring. It is not a question here of seeking approval or compliments, but only of allowing our most beautiful feeling to express itself, that of basic joy, which can end up involving others.

Often the older people themselves possess the strength of the moose and can therefore encourage the younger ones and advise them on how to use their courage and achieve success.

They know when it is appropriate to be kind and friendly and when it is necessary to give vent to their righteous anger. The moose shows how important it is to know how to be brave and to appreciate the results obtained as well as it is necessary to learn how to praise and encourage others because from this anyone can benefit.

Eagle

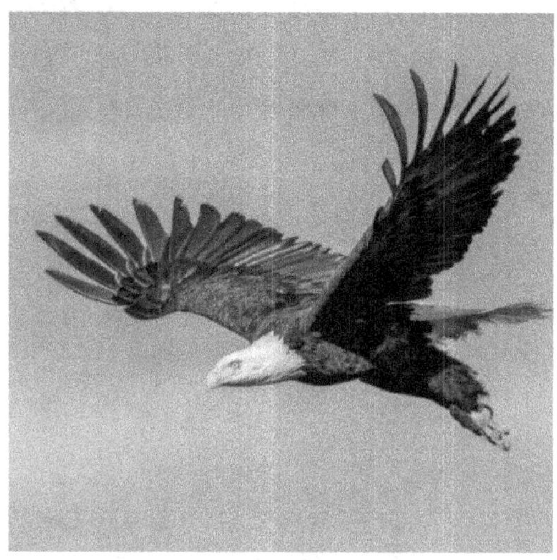

It is said that the Eagle flies higher than all birds and can get close to the Creator so as to bring him the messages and prayers of the people.

"The eagle is the messenger of the Creator, stated Alvin Manitopyes." The eagle symbolizes the love the Creator has for the North American Indian people .... the eagle is the most spiritually evolved of all animals and birds.

It is the messenger between the Indian people and the Creator. It is a very sacred bird, Manitopyes said. (Eagles) have a lot of courage.." This is why it is a great honour to earn an eagle feather. "Finding an eagle feather is a gift or blessing, Manitopyes explained, and an affirmation of one's spiritual experience."

The greatest representative of the divine force, the Great Spirit, among American Indian myths and legends has always been the eagle, an animal with strong royal connotations with the power to overpower the material world and all that inhabits it. As it hovers in the sky it is able to have a detached and spiritual vision of the human events because it is not influenced by them, this is one of the characteristics of the eagle but it can also be a representative of the negative side of the character of the person who owns the totem of the eagle because it will be too cold and detached in respect to what will happen around him/her in his/her life.

This animal totem, however, has the prerogative of being able to see the plot of existence in a wider and more expanded sense, understanding how the events will unfold before they take place in everyday life, the eagle can also see the shadow that is hidden in the events without which nothing can be learned in this life since without evil there could not be good and vice versa. In order to obtain the strength of the eagle it is necessary to reach the trust in the divine will or in the laws of existence where a man can get it only through the hard trials of life and great strength of mind.

Since the beginning of time the great shamans of the tribes have always used eagle feathers to help heal people, to indicate the courage that the warrior needs to face battle as well as life. Learn to have the courage to really see the things of life without fear to recognize the truth, use the light of the eagle spirit to look from above the events drawing wisdom and knowledge.

Armadillo

This animal has an armor that allows him to defend himself from all predators, which covers him like a warm and safe "blanket", for this reason who owns the animal totem of the armadillo must understand how he tends to close himself to others when he feels threatened, putting his head between his legs and closing the ball trying to avoid direct confrontation with those who press him but at the same time trying to escape from the situation that he does not like literally rolling away from the problem.

This attitude of the armadillo puts him in the situation of being able to decide what he wants to see present in his life as well as what he does not want to see, which sometimes can also be useful to the protégé of the armadillo the ability to slide off his shoulders many situations that would make anyone explode, but at the same time it also puts him in the situation of passing for a person who does not care about others or their protests or words.

The armadillo was often depicted on medicine shields designed for what the wearer wanted to achieve as another great potential of this totem animal is the fact that it continues tirelessly towards its goals not caring about any obstacles or attacks. This protective armor of the armadillo prevents those who have this totem from committing actions that we really do not want to generate, but at the same time allows us to stay in our shell from the demands of others: it can free you from the habit of always saying yes and recognize whether the situation in which you are hunting is good or bad for yourself.

Buffalo

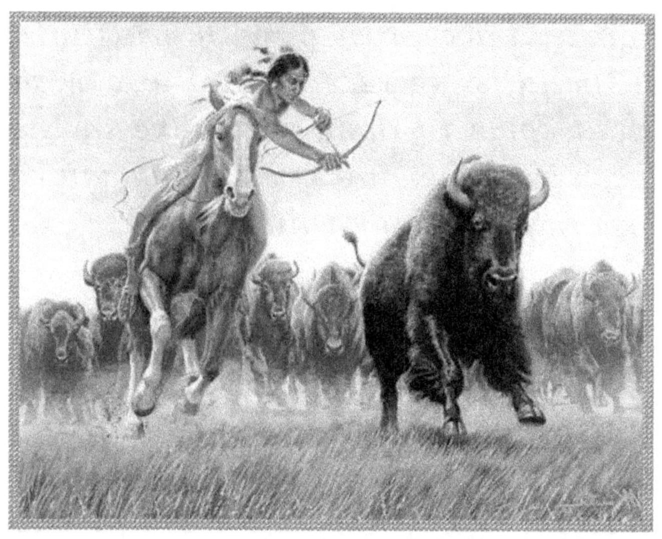

For American Indians the fact that there were millions of bison automatically meant the fact that the abundance would never end, until the arrival of the white man of course, because they drew not only sustenance from the meat of bison but also useful items for survival such as warm furs for cold winters, sinew to make strings for bows so they could hunt and fight, bones to be used to build tools of various kinds or to be used in sacred rites, fat for lamps to illuminate the tents and the night if needed, and much more.

If after the rites or prayers of the tribe or even personal appeared a white bison they thought that their requests would be granted because the white bison was the symbol of Wanca Tanka the sacred buffalo that was recognized as the form of the Great Spirit or Supreme God that supported them in everyday life, punishing them if necessary, gave them his own life to allow them to live and at the same time had also created them.

From a legend we read that a female white bison brought as a gift a sacred pipe to human beings, where in the tobacco that would be used were united all the forces of nature that would bring the prayers of the people to the spirits making visible the desires of the Indians to the divinity that would welcome and fulfill them. The bison teaches that all things are present in abundance when we learn to respect them and accept them with gratitude, because it is essential to appreciate all the gifts we receive and also wish others that the kingdom of Wanca Tanka come to them a bit like in the Catholic tradition of the bible, also the bison shows us that everything can be obtained but only with the help of the Great Spirit of the white bison.

Dog

In every human society the dog is an animal that represents fidelity, reliability, since there is an atavistic connection between dog and human, perhaps also due to the fact that in prehistoric times, when man was able to domesticate this type of animal, a deeper bond than we think was created between our race and his. Even if the owner treats his dog with violence, it does not escape but always returns to obey the will of his "boss" always reciprocating with love and loyalty, even sacrificing his own life, despite the unfair treatment suffered.

For the American Indians the dog is the guardian of the sacred places or of the secret ones, guardian of the knowledge, of the compassion, teaches to overlook many injustices, that one can suffer in life: from the dog one can learn these qualities, learning to be faithful not only towards others, but also towards oneself.

Beaver

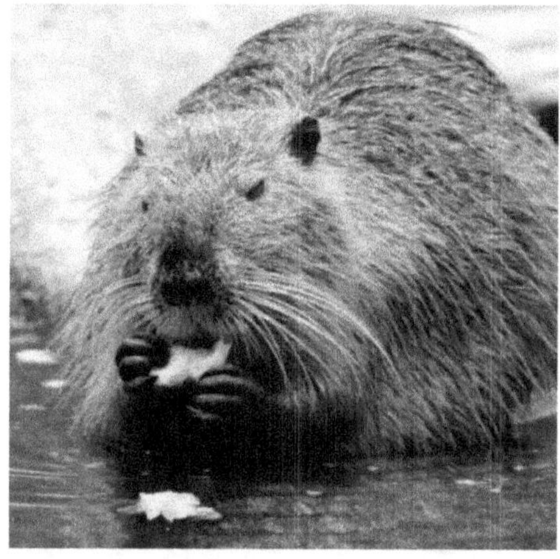

Many Indians believed that beavers could think like humans, had their own laws and language, and were directed by their own chief. Many stories and songs were made about beavers.

The beaver is a very intelligent animal proof of this is the fact that its engineering constructions often put even the best human engineers to shame, it also has an excellent sense of cooperation.

Who has the totem of the beaver has the strength and mental ability to achieve his dreams and desires by collaborating with others, always ready to act to defend himself with his teeth against those who want to prevent him from progressing according to his plans and his will. If we find ourselves in the situation of having a problem that we are unable to remedy, we can evoke the strength of the beaver so as to resonate with its abilities and find a way out of the problem or some information that will help us to overcome the obstacle.

The beaver's way of acting seems to work with the axiom "When you close a door there is always another way to proceed in life". Following his teaching, in fact, we should never get to the point of closing possibilities for ourselves. When the beaver appears to you in a dream, this can mean to make an old wish come true, or to finally bring to fruition an old project.

Horse

Introduced among the Indians by the Spanish at the beginning of the 16th century, the horse soon became fundamental, a true catalyst and essential element of the new culture of the Great Plains.

The horse became a very important part of all Plains Indian tribes. Every family owned at least one and every person learned to ride at a very young age.

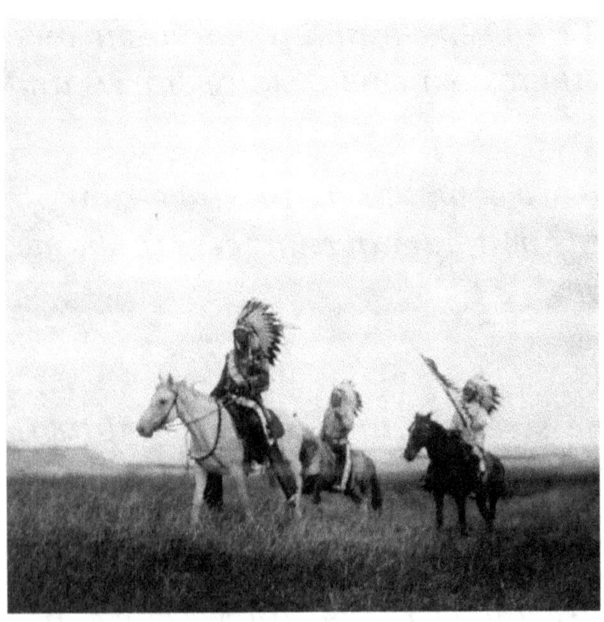

The horse that had made possible the new way of life, became the dominant symbol of wealth prestige in honour as well as the main reason for raids and intertribal wars.

The ancestral force of the earth, the most atavistic emotions that guide the lives of living beings, which is the basis of any desire that is not driven by high ideals but by the simple desire to survive to exist, but also the power to deal with the world beyond and for this reason it was often considered very important for those who became shaman, coming to recognize their ceremonial drum as it was "his horse" with which to move in other worlds to accomplish the missions that were necessary to bring health or other needs.

The horse was the first animal totem of the Indian civilization, something that has remained even in the civilization of the whites so much so that the name of the horse is used to describe the power of the engine as in the Mustang: if you want to experience for once in your life the sense of freedom that almost nothing can give the world, just ride a horse allowing yourself to be possessed by the feeling that it transmits to your rider, that force that the beating of the hooves beating on the ground is transmitted to those who ride, feeling penetrated by a magical force and omnipotent.

The teaching that the horse gives us is that power or strength cannot be obtained only by wanting them, but that they will be achieved only by those who show respect and are ready to take responsibility. Just as the horse carries the rider on its back, so whoever owns the totem of the horse carries the responsibility of his own situation on his own.

The strength symbolized by the horse is wisdom, the ability to remember the steps taken during life and to understand the meaning of them in previous lives, in fact the real power is made of strength applied with wisdom and the ways to achieve this are love, compassion and the ability to share with others their knowledge and their achievements. Even more important is to avoid blocking the way for yourself with your ego.

Deer

According to American Indian tribes, the deer represents friendship and love linked to the desire that consumes and drives the atavistic desires that do not allow to stop what you feel but to reach the purpose of mating even risking death in the attempt.

The physiognomy of the deer, according to native teachings, seems to indicate that the deer is not so careful to recognize the white or the black part, but it penetrates both to reach the goal using what it knows for its own purposes. The love that the deer is able to generate has the power to heal any past or present wound in the person who is the object of its attention, trying to get the person who is passing through bad waters out of trouble.

If the deer shows up in our dreams, it brings the message to love others in spite of character flaws or actions that are not exactly positive towards us, leaving aside our expectations since no one should be forced to be what they are not, but only loved for what they are.

Another lesson we can learn from the deer is to keep intact our spiritual attitude, always direct it towards the good without being influenced by negative people or situations, letting them melt in the air by themselves, keeping friendly and trustful even in the most difficult situations, only in this way the divine energy will be open.

Swan

The animal totem of the swan symbolizes the ability to receive the good fortune brought by changes, submitting its will to that of the Great Spirit, not opposing the evolution but following the vicissitudes almost like a leaf carried by the current of the stream.

In fact, it is born as an ugly chick but over time it turns into a regal swan of enormous beauty, leaving what was the world of appearances to enter the new reality that surrounds it in a continuous whirlwind of positive changes, even coming to predict the future, qualities that possess those who have the animal totem of the swan, because they are completely able to accept without mental or spiritual blocks the will of the divine that explicates in its various intricate designs of existence.

The swan teaches us to bring our consciousness into harmony with all levels of being and to carefully develop our intuition: this helps us to achieve the ability to see into the future.

Owl

The symbol of magic, mystery and prescience par excellence in American Indian cultures is the owl that was also defined as "the eagle of the night", able to see beyond normal human limits, even though the darkness the owl feels at ease, moving in complete silence as if it became part of the environment.

Those who possess the energy of the owl are often interested in esotericism, magic, occultism, in all those "strange" and mysterious sciences that normally people are not interested in, it also seems that it is impossible to keep a secret in their presence because they are able to know things in an almost paranormal way or they can perceive other people's thoughts without problems, even if for them it is normal, for other people those who do not possess the energy of the owl bring a lot of reverence and fear.

The owl is the bird of wisdom, because it is able to see and hear things that escape other animals, helping to recognize the truth and interpret the directions of destiny.

Hummingbirds

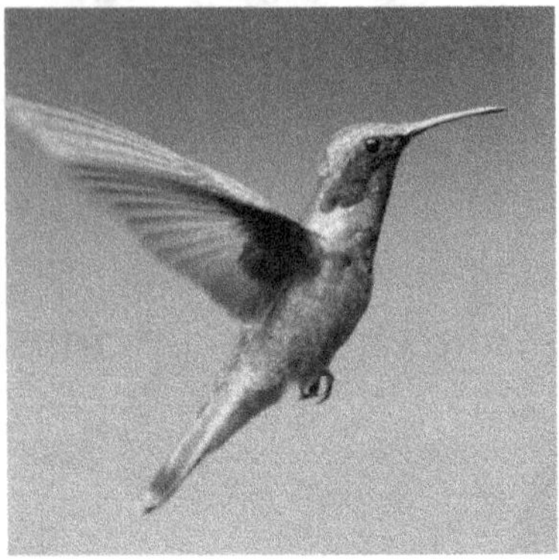

The totem of the hummingbird represents the joy of living and the love for life, happiness despite everything, the power to make the spirit fly despite difficulties. It represents the ability to be completely grafted in the nature that surrounds him and in all the situations that happen around him but at the same time he is also very concentrated towards possible elements of danger or that can disturb him in that case he escapes in a flash from them avoiding every problem or difficulty he can leave behind.

When we talk about healing power referring to some totems we talk about "medicine" that is a power or a mental attitude that possesses the cure to another attitude, however wrong for the harmony of life, that the subject tends to have towards existence. The medicine of the hummingbird are joy and love that must be given to who is near the subject affected by the power of this totem.

Rabbit

Fear finds its true form in the totem rabbit because it is an extremely fearful and cautious animal, always afraid of anything, any noise or even just the suspicion that there may be a danger, always afraid of the idea that the lynx or a coyote can eat him or even other fierce animals: in practice he is afraid of everything around him and with this thought he acts in the world often preferring to remain in the third floor, always hidden from the view of others, sometimes even complaining that others do not care about him but not realizing that his own fear generates this fact, since he instinctively hides from the eyes and interest of others since invariably his fears are realized in concrete facts that strengthen his instinct to escape.

If you are interested in this animal totem, try as much as possible to always think negatively, try to see things for what they are without exaggerating or negating them if reality does not really have negative sides. It can be asserted almost with certainty of denial that it is the totem animal of those who suffer from hypochondria (fear of always being on the verge of dying for who knows what disease sometimes even invented, just read the work of Molière's imaginary sick) otherwise you will be able to "be satisfied" because it will happen just what you are afraid of, to make you learn that what you think strongly you end up attracting, exactly as the Universal Spiritual Law states.

Everyone is primarily responsible for the things that happen to him, personal responsibility first.

Crow

According to the legends of American Indians the crow was the holder of the great mysteries often invoked by shamans in sacred ceremonies where they asked for advice for the tribe or in the case of propitiatory rituals in hunting. According to the myths of the natives it would be the only animal that can contravene the laws of the physical world transforming itself into other animals or that can take advantage of the gift of ubiquity.

Its knowledge is absolute because it sees along the space-time timeline without fail because the crow exists in a reality where time has no meaning exactly as it could happen in the stories of the great enlightened ones who lived in a timeless time. In this timeless substance, good and evil, light and darkness join together, losing themselves and interpenetrating, therefore the dualisms of matter disappear, leaving pure truth without hypocrisy or falsehood.

Some people considered the crow as a negative animal bearer of ominous omens, but in truth it announces that all the creation is created by the woman and by the sacred generating energy, here is that the real and supreme truth not obscured by false dogmas or limiting laws comes to the light of the mind to overcome the obstacles of mental understanding.

Those who are possessed by the energy of the crow must increase their efforts to be always consistent with the discoveries of which they are informed and live in reality through the truth that they possess and that they have learned to know directly, trying to make their inner guidance stronger and stronger, changing shape in the identity that they might have in the future.

Coyote

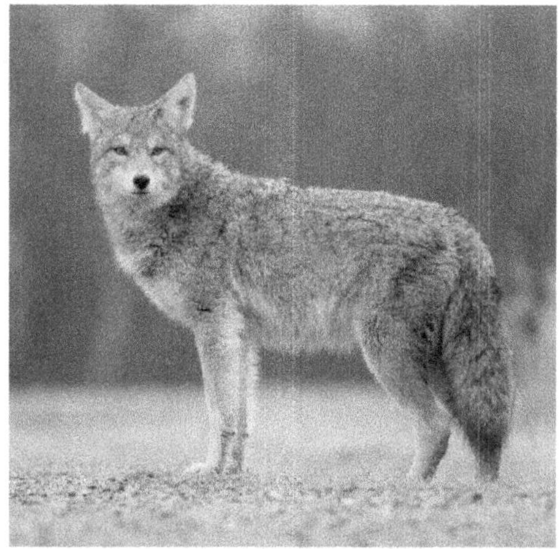

In all the traditions of the world there is a being "joker" and treacherous who enjoys or seems to enjoy doing evil or create strife or problems to the poor mortals here is the coyote is one of these only that belongs to the tradition of thousands of American Indians, but just like all the traditions I mentioned, it is immensely sacred because the Coyote represents chaos and its incessant work to generate new possibilities.

He always falls in his own traps and then he manages to get out every time still unharmed as a phoenix rising from its own ashes, not learning from his own mistakes he often falls into the same negative patterns of action causing the same identical problems. The coyote has the peculiarity of being able to live for the day, he doesn't work easily, he tries to take advantage of any and all opportunities as soon as he has the chance, working as little as possible using what life allows him to use to stay alive.

If you belong to this type of energy and your animal totem is the Coyote, you will often find yourself playing the clown and it will always seem that you end up in the most difficult and strange situations without having the slightest intention: at this point know that the only way for you to overcome the problem will be to learn to laugh at you and the situation without letting you demotivate or fall into depression. the coyote is that totem that represents our dark inner part that often unconsciously guides our steps making us find ourselves in adverse situations but only to make you get to know yourself better and take life with greater lightness.

Dolphin

The lesson of the dolphin is to make us learn to breathe, because the breath represents the union of the spirit with the physical body, the life that enters and leaves every living being and therefore the cyclic process of life-death. Changing the respiratory rhythm, we can visit the worlds beyond physicality, those of the afterlife, where mysterious and superior beings to modern man reside.

The Great Spirit, God, communicates with all of us through the breath, just as the breath can actually control emotions and physical reactions or its functionality as yogis well know. Those who have the power of the dolphin can act as intermediaries with spiritual realities and humans.

Peculiarities of the dolphin are to teach how to overcome the vicissitudes of life with happiness and harmony without being sunk by heavy thoughts or obstacles and difficulties on the path of life, following their own path guided by the heart and instinct almost childlike. If you have the dolphin in your totem try to consciously free yourself from all the weights and impediments by projecting them outside your body and your being through exhalation!

Weasel

The weasel is the totem that can tell us what is hidden behind the mask that others want us to see to hide their real intentions or that we ourselves put on to hide some part of us that we do not fully accept. According to tradition the weasel can with little information perceive or understand what is going to be generated in a situation and for this reason there were many warriors who wore weasel skins.

Those who possess the power of the weasel is often underestimated because they are people who prefer confidentiality and for this reason the common people not knowing everything about these objects think that they are not worth much because they do not give airs of greatness as it is common in society. Instead, the subjects guided by the power of the weasel are excellent in business thanks to their acumen and their sagacity they are able to anticipate the opponents preceding them and defeating them before they can respond.

However, the weasel is a rather difficult totem animal because almost always these subjects feel responsible for the fact that they perceive things that come true while they can only perceive the facts before they happen, they don't make them happen and often end up closing themselves to society and the world, becoming loners who don't want to know about people because they know too much about reality and they don't let themselves be guided towards easy ideals or arguments without art or part.

Hawk

The hawk is the messenger of the other totem animals, exactly as in many other cultures in the world, the hawk has the power to communicate the will of the divinity or to warn if events are going to happen, but they are not yet recognized as positive or negative, and for this reason the wisdom of the hawk suggests to keep eyes open to evaluate the situation and understand what to expect from the events, in order to act with courage if necessary.

The hawk totem suggests to open to the gifts of life that are prepared by the Great Spirit, God, who has everything ready for each of us but if we do not open and prepare to enjoy these gifts we will not be able to get anything.

Exactly as the hawk possesses a sharp sight and prefers to observe before choosing the moment to act by observing every detail that surrounds it. If you happen to hear the squeak of a hawk inwardly, carefully observe things from a broader perspective in order to fully understand the meaning of its warning.

Ant

In the ant totem there are many qualities such as great physical strength, aggressiveness in case of need, being generous and even sacrificing their lives for their group, being precise and hard worker as well as tireless.

Patience and resistance are the most incisive characters of the ant that is able to wait patiently for hours before going on the counterattack or waiting to receive orders, without ever giving up or giving up the fight by getting torn to pieces if necessary for the survival of the anthill.

The teaching of the ant says that you can get what you want and need with hard work, a symbol of the deepest confidence knows that after all his efforts will be satisfied with the gift that he wanted and earned with the sweat of his brow. The ant serves the common good, that of society or of the family of the group, in short, ready to sacrifice his own for the greater good.

Dragonfly

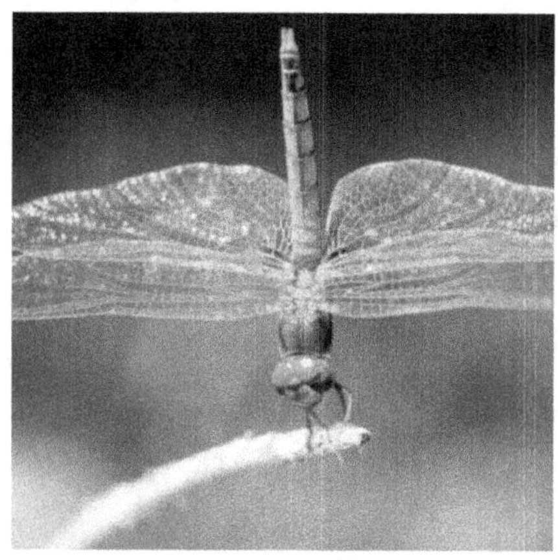

Despite it is not a real animal because it belongs to insects, dragonflies were often identified as totems even though any living being can become the symbol of one's interiority and it does not necessarily have to belong to the category of mammals or similar in order to have access to it.

The dragonfly symbolizes change and illusions, connected to magic and illusion because of its iridescent body teaches us that reality in truth is not real and for this we must appreciate the gift of the sacred "dream" as the Australian aborigines call it, we must overcome the illusions on which we base our lives in order to perceive the truth in everyday things. If you want to make important changes, it is appropriate to evoke the energy of the dragonfly.

Lynx

The keepers of the secrets of nature and the various totems are several depending on the traditions and cultures of the American Indian tribes and this of the lynx is one of them, since it holds the secrets of the totems, knowing all the secrets and ancient mysteries now lost and forgotten. The silence characterizes it because it is what the lynx is looking for, solitude and silence to live beyond the schemes of ordinary mortals and nature, in continuous *flow with the existence free from any constraint it moves without others can understand its essence or how much it can know.*

If the lynx appears in your dreams means that a secret is hidden and you have to do everything to know it because it affects your personal freedom or your lifestyle: if you belong to the energy of the lynx then you are an individual with a lot of inner light, you are seers and love introspection, with which you can find your true self and your true identity, while those who know you or around you can never understand who you are or what you are thinking.

Those belonging to the lynx totem know how to expose the liars or double-crossers and also find their own unknown sides. They will also know how to recognize with certainty the techniques of self-deception that everyone uses on a daily basis.

The only way to come into possession of some of the lynx's knowledge is to pay her properly to reveal it, according to the custom of shamans and prophets. This custom is in fact part of their tradition and is based on the principle of mutual exchange of energies.

Otter

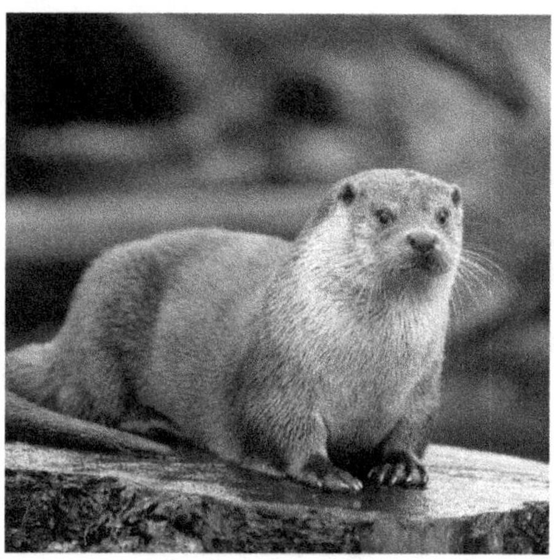

The totem of the otter possesses the feminine energy which can be defined passive, nourishing, which takes care of others, it is therefore part of the elements of earth and water where the first represents the highest degree of passivity while the second possesses a part of the active principle because it moves from a certain point of view, following gravity by letting itself fall - it would be better to say so - going down to the valley.

The otter is a joyful and playful animal in fact it spends most of the day playing with its young and cleaning or feeding them, it never attacks first but if it must it defends itself relentlessly. The otter is an animal with a very pronounced curiosity and approaches every new situation with openness and without negative mental schemes. This is a very beautiful thing, but it often gets her into trouble because she finds herself involved in problems that she would have preferred not to know.

The ideal of woman among American Indian tribes was represented by the weasel, that is slender and very flirtatious with men, a mixture of fake shyness and great sweetness. This totem teaches that being a woman has nothing to do with jealousy and mistrust, but instead is synonymous with joy and sincerity, is the strength of generosity, of sharing what you have with others. Individuals endowed with the energy of the otter seek free love without false limits and without power plays.

They let themselves be carried along by the river of life without regard or attachment to material possessions. This is the powerful receptive force of women.

Wolf

The wolf is related, in the Indian tradition, with the star Sirius in the constellation of Leo, from which, according to legend, came the masters of antiquity.

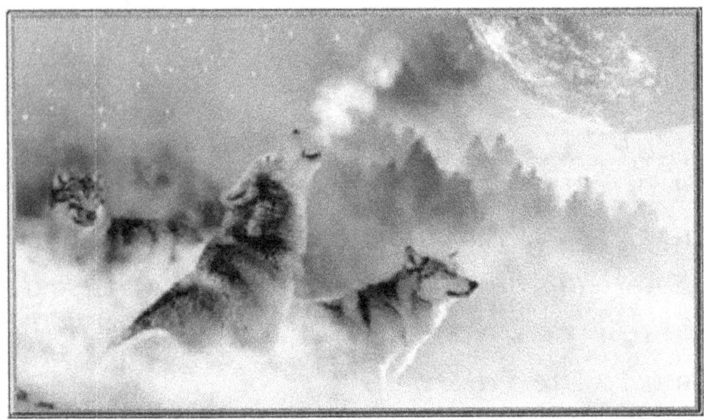

In fact, the wolf is also considered a master, who after a long wanderings returns to his pack to report his observations and experiences.

He lives strictly within the family, but without giving up his independence. He chooses a companion to whom he will remain faithful for the rest of his life.

Howling at the moon, he rejoins its strength, its spiritual energy and the power of the unconscious, the way to knowledge.

The wolf can give us the energy to teach others, to help them better understand life and find their own way.

Using the strength of the wolf we can succeed in regaining contact with our inner teacher.

The star of Sirius finds many contacts with the totem of the wolf in the American Indian tradition, present in the constellation of Leo, from where the sacred celestial masters who indoctrinated the human society of the Indians of antiquity came from. The wolf is recognized as an inner master who after a period of inner research returns to the tribe to bring back and pass on what he has learned from his research and his experiences.

The wolf is extremely tied to his family and obeys to a rigid bureaucratic procedure made of levels and recognition of respect where each member has special duties and peculiarities and for this reason he is questioned in case of need, but he never gives up his personal freedom. If the wolf finds a suitable mate, he remains faithful to her all his life: this totem represents the strength of the unconscious, the darkness where the monsters of the psyche hide, but also the inner knowledge of what is called "guardian of the threshold" in many esoteric traditions.

The wolf can give us the energy to teach others, to help them better understand life and find their own s

Opossum

This totem animal is specialized in strategy, but when his aims are not successful he pretends to be dead, so as to confuse the animal from which he is fleeing or against which he is fighting that actually remains rather confused and usually leaves him alone.

Usually it is difficult to see an opossum fighting with nails and teeth even if it is equipped with them, it prefers to pass for dead or escape through this cunning tactic rather than risk losing its life unnecessarily, it even comes to smell like a corpse just to pass for dead.

The possum's teaching is the use of rationality and intuition united in a single weapon to be able to find solutions to the problems and vicissitudes of life. Even a warrior can take advantage of the wisdom and technique of the possum by using surprise and confusing the enemy so that the latter thinks he has a superiority in numbers or strength. Victory in the end depends on the best strategy, and the possum shows precisely how important it is to refine the ability to pretend and surprise.

Bear

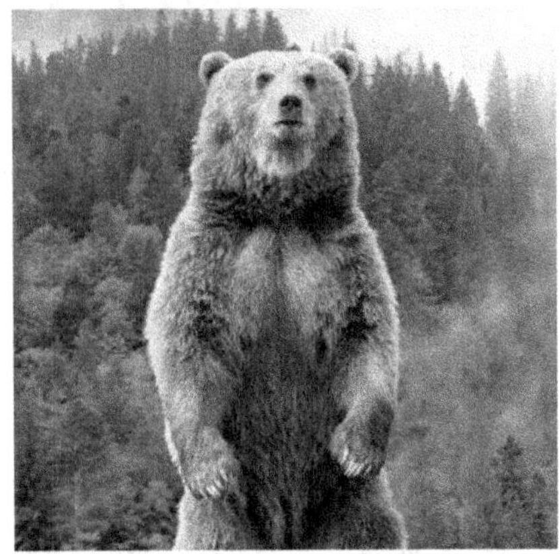

The bear was respected and admired for its strength and courage. The Indians hunted it for its meat and especially for its fat, which they stored in bags. Winter clothing and moccasins were made from bear skins.

Bow strings were made from twisted bear gut laces as well as sinew, rawhide, and woven plant fibres. Bear oil was applied to the hair and mixed with paint. The bear's claws were highly valued. Some peoples had the bear as their totem and did not kill it.

The bear is the most quoted totem animal in American Indian traditions, as it represents the primordial force of ferocity when it has to fight but also introspection, the search in the cave where one spends the winter, symbolically a period of stasis where one stops from the normal habits of society to look for the answers to the questions of life or to the questions about one's own existence, a period that can also be used to try to digest and *therefore overcome events that have devastated us or put us out of balance inside so that we can go back to acting correctly instead of going on without strength and without guides.*

The lesson of the bear shows us how it is extremely important to find time every now and then to take stock of the situation and think about our future directions, because only through calm, we can manage to listen to the voice of our innermost being, which can give us the answers to all our questions or the solution to all our problems.

Bat

The totem of the bat indicates, contrary to the normal negative meaning given by the castrating Catholic religion, rebirth in a broad sense, since it prefers to stay in holes and dark recesses as are the graves, resting upside down as only he knows how to do, a position that represents that of the unborn child before his coming into the world. Usually the bat is worshipped only in Central America where the Aztec and Mayan cultures had a primary role.

This animal totem indicates the ritual and symbolic death that those who undertake the path of shamanism must overcome to return another person from the afterlife and be able to become a reference and a link for others of his tribe. The initiatory death is present in many cultures of esoteric type where those who must be initiated must pass through the stage of personal death in order to be reborn inwardly and be able to see things in a broader way and without preconceptions, in short, must die the rational mind to bring out his true superior mind because as Osho said "the mind ... mind".

The initiation trials have always been very hard to the limit of madness just see that in some tribes when the chosen one had to be initiated was buried in a coffin for a night, something that would drive anyone crazy but only the future shaman would return to earth changed inside into something superior.

If a bat appears in your dream you must try to break away from the habitual things or even it could mean that your lifestyle no longer suits you and it is time that you start thinking about changing things.

Porcupine

The hedgehog has a friendly and non-violent character, in fact for this reason it is placed inside the medicine wheel in the place called "the innocent child", if someone dares to attack it, it will be enough to show its thorns to make the aggressor desist from continuing.

A person under the hedgehog possesses characteristics such as faith, trust, two forces that put together are very powerful for those who possess them and know how to use them, in fact it is enough to think about the famous saying that "faith also moves mountains" to understand what a person can do if he is able to have enough faith inside himself.

The totem of the hedgehog teaches us to remain open to those who stand in front of us, finding in every day new stimulus in the wonders of life, letting go of the limitations dictated by excessive seriousness, remaining as children who are able to remain amazed by a nothing or who still believe in the stories that the elders often tell them about strange beings and magical fairy.

Friendliness and openness to others help to open hearts and share joy and love with them.

Puma

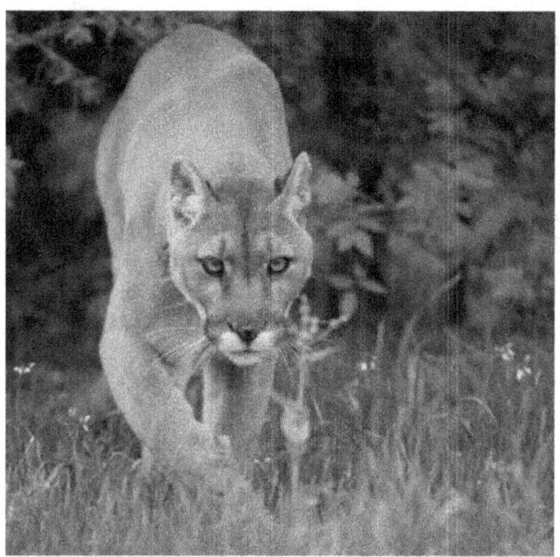

The mountain lion known as puma symbolizes the pure strength of the mountain and of what is hidden from everyone's sight because it is famous for its sudden and studied ambushes towards those who unwisely enter its territory.

It is a force that is said to be used for the good by Indian chiefs and wise men of the tribes but it can also be used for one's own purposes and desires, in this case it is often used badly and improperly because it only helps one's ego to have what it desires even though a bit of healthy selfishness is not wrong. By carefully observing the puma moving we can appreciate its sinuosity and elegant movements difficult to recognize in a big cat like this, which indicates how the union of its three main bodies (physical body, mind and spirit) can act when they move in unison and with the natural flow of events.

The puma urges us to hold on to our deepest beliefs and to always stick to the truth: these are the qualities that characterize a person who can lead or guide others. Obtaining a position of leadership involves great difficulties, for example, it will be very difficult to always please everyone, or maintain peace in the tribe for a long time.

When you have a lot of strength, in addition to the difficulties of managing this, you must also manage not to be manipulated by external subjects or events that are not directly related to you, otherwise you end up hurting those you wanted to help or defend.

A man with the energy of the puma must avoid showing fear or too fragile and must be ready to take on great responsibility, also should try to maintain a certain respectful detachment from his peers.

Skunk

The skunk has a lot of self-confidence in fact in its actions it always shows how the tranquillity and security of a creature that is aware of its strength and its limits can give the correct directions to move properly in life. Although she doesn't possess any really dangerous weapon of defense, she instills a reverential fear in men, if only for the horrible stench spray that she possesses and directs towards those who disturb her.

People led by the strength of the skunk generally possess a lot of charisma, attracting others of their kind almost like human magnets or like the intense smell of the skunk that has an attractive effect on other individuals of the species.

This skunk can teach us to find our completeness by developing a healthy dose of pride and self-love, we can then automatically attract people of our own species and energetically reject those who have nothing in common with us or who only intend to use us for their own purposes.

Spider

Although the spider is not an animal but an arachnid is commonly recognized as a being who weaves the web that the Vikings and Celts called Wird or destiny, through which lucid dreams of humans are manifested in our reality building what surrounds us and interacts with all of us.

The spider represents the infinite without time or space that devours those who have come to the end of their lives, closing them in their cocoon to preserve the idea that they had of themselves and then feed on it, destroying them exactly as time destroys everything in the course of the endless existence of the infinite lives of every being. The number four doubled indicates both the four winds and the four celestial directions.

If people feel like victims caught in this web they have not yet understood the meaning of the lesson and remain imprisoned in a false reality that they cannot change. The lesson of the spider is that every being is responsible for the events of their lives and that it is necessary not to get lost in the falsehoods of their own senses. The spider also symbolizes the characters of writing.

The spirit hunter acts in this exact way capturing the nightmares generated by our own mind to allow the dreamer to continue to dream only true things not necessarily beautiful to his mind.

Toad

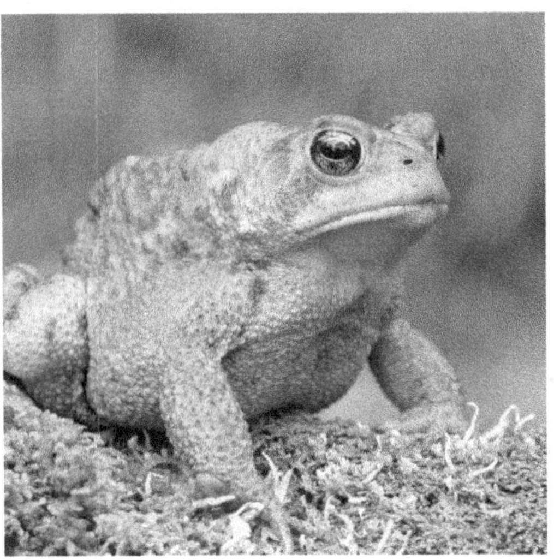

The toad belongs to the element of water and to the purifying force of rain and is somehow present in all initiatory rites centered on the element of water was also used to evoke rain in times of dryness often using objects carved in the shape of toads rubbed with a stick of the same material that produced the sound of toads when they inhabit the ponds in the hope that the sympathetic magic could help the rain to arrive in the region that suffered thirst.

Individuals endowed with the strength of the toad are often skilled mediums or healers, able to exorcise the place they are in, ridding a house of malignant entities, or even free a sick person from their pains. The toad also announces the beginning of a process of transformation or a new phase of life.

If a toad appears to you in a dream, it is a sign that the time has come to take a break and observe yourself inside, purifying you from every thought or wrong attitude, or freeing you from a situation of stagnation that no longer has anything positive for your existence.

Squirrel

The squirrel always thinks about the dark times and for this reason he stores seeds and anything else that may serve him to survive hiding his "treasures" throughout the woods near his burrow making a mental map of the places where he buries or simply blocks in some crevice of the acorns of which he feeds but ends up forgetting some that for this reason will become part of the for this reason they will become part of the new part of the forest, growing into new trees born from the acorns that manage to survive the winter, a sign that the squirrel often sows and then ends up not caring about the fruits that his actions can bring to others, but in his disinterest he improves the world in which he lives without realizing it.

The squirrel is also famous for being an animal full of energy, always active and intent on working to improve his situation, fast in his movements as well as in his thoughts that no one can divert for more than a few moments, because he has great power of adaptation which allows him to act quickly to changes, finding particularly ingenious solutions to the obstacles that are placed in front of him. If you dream of a squirrel you have to prepare for the future by organizing yourself in the face of big changes, getting rid of unnecessary burdens and situations that no longer serve you.

Snake

In all initiatory traditions and cultures that had contact with the snake it represents infinity, the cycle of life and death, rebirth, the sacred wheel is already a stylized snake, the continuous change of events in relation to actions and nature.

Connected to the snake there are symbols related to sexuality, creation, soul, immortality, therefore finding people who have this kind of energy on their side is immensely difficult because it leads to have access to an energy close to divinity that hardly a human being could ever "control" or be guided by in a balanced way, but also because in order to have this honour among the experiences that these people have to go through there is to come in contact with poisons without being damaged by transforming these substances in other more assimilable ones.

The snake is a creature connected to the element of fire: at the level of the body this generates passion and desire, but at the spiritual level it leads to access the Great Spirit and to realize the wisdom that includes everything. If the snake appears in your dreams it means that you must begin to change yourself, leaving the old to access new levels of personal consciousness.

Turkey

The turkey represents an animal that not many would expect to be recognized as a great warrior and fighting animal but is generally branded as a passive and stupid animal, which is not true. It represents the fast and fleeting passing of one's possessions, therefore it teaches us that it is useless to accumulate more than we need, inviting us to sacrifice the surplus to others so that they can live better tasting the flavor of life.

Who has this kind of energy tends to act for the good of others and society in an altruistic way, which arises from the fact of recognizing that the Great Spirit is present and alive in every living being and that there is a universal law that asserts that as we give to others, others will give to us one day.

The teaching of the turkey is therefore the sharing in fact it is used as a symbol of sharing that the Indians, still unaware of how things would go with the white Quakers, did with the newcomers who were in a moment of food difficulty and from that day we celebrate Thanksgiving in America. If you dream of a turkey can mean, among other things that you will receive an unexpected gift.

Turtle

The turtle is an important animal. It was used as a calendar and teaches an important lesson. All turtles have 13 sections on the upper back that represent the 13 moons and all have 28 sections surrounding the lower part of the upper shell that represents the number of days in each moon. The top of the curved shell represents the universe. The lower part of the shell represents the earth.

The turtle represents the power of our Mother Earth, who warns us not to rush too suddenly into our choices but to take our time to reason and think properly before implementing our wills, waiting for the right time to implement the right actions.

The turtle teaches us to let events bring about the opportunities we need so as to follow the flow of life instead of fighting against it, thus saving precious energies and obtaining more easily what we desire, just as the turtle lets the sun warm and enliven its eggs.

The turtle also teaches us to think a lot before letting others know our points of view and our thoughts so as to avoid mistakes dictated by haste keeping our feet firmly planted in the stable ground, avoiding not understanding the reality of situations.

Badger

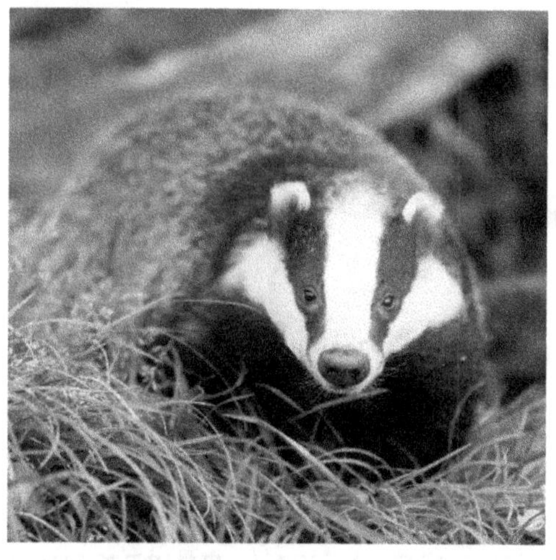

The teaching of the Badger is how to use creativity and aggression at the exact moment when one is needed rather than the other, in fact every animal readily avoids having to deal with this animal knowing what he would be up against if he were to get something wrong.

The badger is the animal-totem of healers and women shamans. A man with the strength of the badger can use his tenacity to heal others because he will not give up even in the most difficult cases insisting until the disease disappears.

The message brought by the badger is to use your anger, to get to change negative or very tangled situations, act relentlessly until the goal is reached. Use your energy to attack, to throw yourself into the fray but without overwhelming those around you and always being careful to keep your balance intact.

Those with badger energy often play the role of the boss, feared by others, but ultimately holding the reins in all situations. When he is in a bad mood, he does not show coldness and meanness, because his strength lies also in being able to show his feelings without caring about the reactions of others. Moreover, he does not know panic and even in the most dangerous situations he always manages to keep his cool and his mind clear.

Mouse

Not many people would like to have the mouse as their totem but I don't understand the subtlety of knowledge that this animal can bring in their life because the mouse demands to observe everything closely, finicky as few, brings us the teaching of looking at things from every angle and then ordering all the knowledge that we can acquire.

He is a born perfectionist who tends to specialize in his interests and needs, although he tends to complicate life with arguments and problems that are often totally useless for real purposes, in fact you can lose sight of the situation as a whole if you insist on wanting to split hairs or even when we observe something too closely we can no longer grasp its overall appearance and its connections with the rest.

People characterized by this energy are generally very fearful, certainly prudent and very accurate in their actions in fact everything they do is orderly and well organized. For them, however, it would be important to be able to dare more and face what they do not know, turn their gaze towards the infinity of the universe and learn to be tolerant.

Fox

The fox has always been recognized as a cunning animal that sneaks into chicken coops to kill chickens, feeding only on their brains, but this sometimes appears more for the mustelids than for the fox. However, the fox represents cunning used for personal purposes to defend its own life or will, especially if used in a negative and selfish way.

The fox hides easily from the eyes of the hunter, blending in with the environment. Its physical agility and its speed have always symbolically represented the speed of thought of cunning and astute people who know how to take advantage of ideal situations to commit their desires without others noticing.

Wapiti

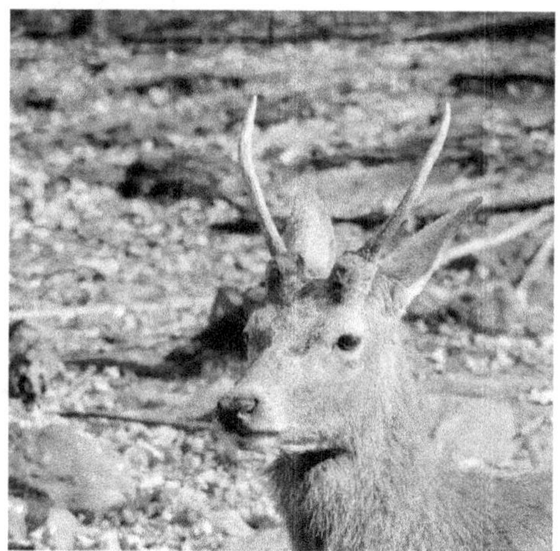

The wapiti is a type of deer that lives especially in Canada and it is very robust, in fact besides the puma only the man can be a danger to his life, its greater advantage is the perfect knowledge of its own limitations and powers so as to know exactly how to act in every situation to face the danger without overcoming them and avoiding to end up in trouble (even if with the man you cannot always run away nor with a hungry puma).

Those who possess this totem are able to reach their goals through their own resistance and intimate knowledge of themselves, being subjects who tend to be very competitive and in need of continuous confirmation of their preparation, they always put themselves to the test in the most disparate occasions and ways.

It symbolizes the feeling of brotherhood between members of the same sex, the mutual support between men can have comforting and encouraging effects through the exchange of experiences and the comparison of their thoughts and personal opinions.

Native American Zodiac Signs

Native American zodiac signs have the names of the animals that are closest to the tribes. As it happens in European culture, even in the villages, the zodiac connects space with the cosmos.

There are those who believe in it and those who do not, those who do not leave home without consulting their horoscope and those who think it's all a fantasy. For Native Americans, animals are an integral part of their lives, which is why they also appear in the symbolism of the signs of the zodiac.

They are associated with the month of birth and are said to have the power to influence values, actions and behaviors, just as in our modern horoscope. All seasons and life cycles of Native Americans are marked by the Indian calendar which is closely linked to the presence of the Great Spirit.

Let's take a look at the zodiac signs together.

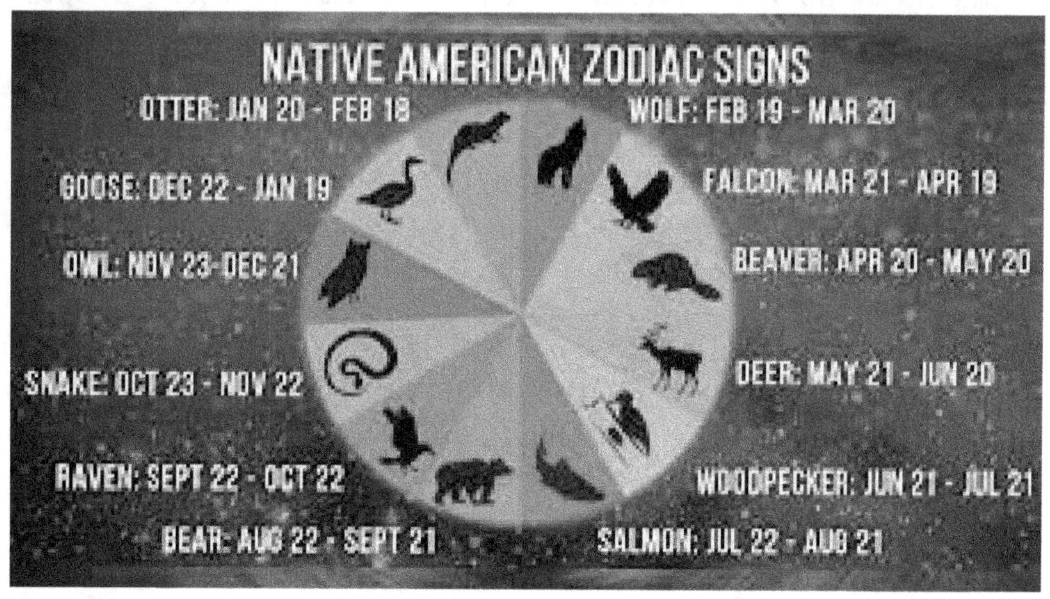

Otter (January 20 - February 18)

Those born under the sign of the otter are optimistic, original and creative people who often behave in an unconventional way. This means that the otter thanks to their intuition and perceptiveness, finds solutions that others would not even imagine. Those born under this sign are caring, understanding, courageous and sincere.

Wolf (February 19 - March 20)

Those born under the sign of the wolf have passion and emotionality. The wolf as we know is able to live in packs and be loyal. According to the Indians, those born under this sign are devoted to philosophy and heart, but at the same time, they are independent people who also love solitude. When it comes to taking care of others, the wolf is ready to give all the support.

Falcon (March 21 - April 19)

Those born under the sign of the hawk know how to keep a cool head when it comes to making important decisions. They are independent people and not from stable ties. Being very pragmatic, this sign does not like to waste time and always remains focused on the goal. Those born under this sign are very good at team sports, but beware they are also very touchy.

Beaver (April 20 - May 20)

Beaver births are tireless workers, but they love to be in charge while adapting to any situation. They are sharp and brilliant with an innate classiness. Unfortunately, the beaver also tends to be very stubborn when they convince themselves that their way is the right way. A little tact wouldn't hurt in certain situations, even if you are on the side of right. Beavers can be loyal, compassionate, helpful and generous. In the emotional field they are very attached to the people they care about and this often leads them to suffer from jealousy.

Deer (May 21 - June 20)

People born in the deer are creative, witty and with a great sense of humor. They bond easily with people, thanks to an innate sympathy and an outgoing nature that sets them apart. The deer, who tends to be a bit cocky, is often focused on himself, tends to be moody and lazy. Thanks to its liveliness, however, is a good partner in any kind of relationship.

Woodpecker (June 21 - July 21)

Woodpecker natives are very sociable and helpful people, true friends. They are empathetic and understanding educators. No other sign is as supportive as the woodpecker. Excellent parents and colleagues. They can sometimes be jealous, prone to anger and very possessive. They tend to be rather frugal but you can always trust them as they are always well organized.

Salmon (July 22 - August 21)

Salmon natives are brave people, always ready to fight for a goal of theirs. Creativity is their strong point, they never lose sight of their goals, they are intuitive and incredibly energetic. Their enthusiasm is almost incurable and is highly contagious, they are always driven by the need to achieve a goal and cross the finish line. In relationships they are calm, generous, stable and sensual.

Brown Bear (August 22 to September 21)

Those born under the sign of the brown bear suffer from a lack of self-confidence so they cannot express their generosity and inner wealth. Pragmatism is their strong point, but in some circumstances the bear is sceptical, lazy and reserved. Humility is also another characteristic of the bear and sometimes, those born under this sign tend to be shy. The bear is cut out for the pedagogical field as it transmits patience those it teaches.

Raven (September 22 to October 22)

Those born under the sign of the Raven are very resourceful, true diplomats, able to alternate between seriousness and humor based on the situations they find themselves in. They possess an energy charge that everyone can count on when new ideas are needed. In some circumstances they can be selfish and inconsistent, but also idealistic and calculating. The positives of the raven are its affable, romantic and posed ways. In relationships crows are intuitive and patient.

Snake (October 23 - November 22)

Those born under the sign of the serpent are real draggers, connected in a spiritual world, not surprisingly it is the traditional sign of shamans. Steady and focused on their goal, they strive almost stubbornly to achieve their goals. Snakes are prone to mystery and darkness, but at the same time people born under this sign can be caring and sensitive. In positive situations they have an exceptional sense of humor, they are very helpful and you can get inspiration from them.

Owl (November 23 - December 21)

Owl births are deeply honest people, bordering on naïve. Curious and intelligent, they are great dreamers, but also very fickle. Those who are part of this sign are people who face life in a determined way and love to explore and adventures. This can, of course, also be dangerous because the owl is sometimes reckless and is often reckless. In difficult situations the owl tends to be aggressive, but because of its eclectic nature it is apt to do many things.

Goose (December 22 - January 19)

The goose born are people who try with great strength and commitment to achieve their goals. Serious and honest, they often fail to be completely communicative with the people they have at their side. Perseverance is what sets this sign in motion, there is nothing holding them back especially when they have family and friends in tow.

Discover your Corresponding Animal

These are the correspondences between zodiac sign and totemic animal:

Aries - Falcon

Taurus - Beaver

Gemini - Deer

Cancer - Woodpecker

Leo - Salmon

Virgo - Brown Bear

Libra - Raven

Scorpio - Snake

Sagittarius - Owl

Capricorn - Goose

Aquarius - Otter

Pisces - Wolf

Full moon of flowers: here's why it was dear to Native Americans

A full moon dear to the natives, with its scents and traditions associated with it. That's why the full moon of May is dedicated to flowers.

May 26th appointment with the moon. Even if the temperatures seem autumn-like, summer is now only a few days away. By now spring is on the wane, with its scents, colors and its ever-present flowers, to which is tied the name of the full moon of May.

Many are the names assigned to this event of the sky, some given by the Native Americans, others by the European tradition. Although today we know every detail about our natural satellite and its cycles, it was not always so.

Every month or so, the moon completes some sort of cycle; these are the so-called lunar phases that describe the appearance it takes on during its motion based on its orientation relative to the Sun. When the Moon moves to the side of the Earth facing the Sun, it shows us its bright face reflecting the sun's rays. This is the time of the full moon.

When all this was not yet known, we relied on our knowledge and beliefs to give a name to astronomical events, such as the phases of the moon.

The one we will admire on May 26 will be the Flower Moon. American tradition also refers to this full moon by the designations Corn Planting Moon or as Milk Moon. For the corn moon, the meaning is immediately understandable. In the second case, milk moon refers to the fact that in May the pastures are rich in good grasses and animals such as cows, goats and sheep, can feed on them. As a result, the milk is very rich in vitamins.

Yana Nashua

Nutrition Native Americans

Food has always been an occasion of friendly entertainment as well as a family meeting or acquaintance for agreements of many kinds, including decisions related to the entry in war of a tribe or a village, for this reason I decided to write a more detailed article including some of the original recipes of Native Americans in order to give a more reasonable and precise description especially to the ones who asserted in the past years that American Indians were almost vegetarian which is not true but they had a varied and very rich diet of meat or fish according to whether they were Indian tribes located along the coast or in the hinterland. American Indian tribes of the north prepared particular dishes, two of which we do not know, such as boiled elk and dog meat which were served on trays made of bark which were thrown away at the end of the meal, the forerunner of today's disposable dishes, only more ecological. The native tribes of the eastern coast ate things that even today are defined as delicacies such as lobsters, seafood as well as various other crustaceans which were steamed or roasted thanks to rudimentary ovens built under the sand and which were covered with glowing stones. Still today in New England this type of cooking is used especially in summertime to cook seafood for local clubs.

Mary Jane Cryan, in a short essay written in 1986, wrote "if, finding yourself visiting the United States, you are invited to a Thanksgiving meal, thank the Indians as well as the hostess. Although modern American cooks today stuff their turkeys and do not use venison, a prestige food of the Indians, the rest of the traditional Thanksgiving menu has not changed much in the last three hundred years. No table would be fully set without cranberry sauce, pumpkin pie, or cornbread, all native foods that the Indians taught the early settlers to prepare and enjoy." Indians did not only leave us particular recipes and traditions but also specific tools such as Simmering pots which are pots for simmering similar to the ones used by Algonkini. An English explorer, Arthur Barlowe, met these tribes around the period from 1580 to 1590 and in the diary of the expedition he wrote: "They use large earthenware pots, so thin that not even the English could do better". Thanks to these pots they cooked a mixture of fruits, meat and fish, (which reminds the Spanish "paella") on a slow and constant fire. Again from Barlowe's diary: "The chief's wife led us into a room where the food was placed on a large table against the wall, like a modern buffet. There we found boiled wheat pudding, game, fish, both boiled and roasted, fresh melons and cooked melons, different kinds of roots, vegetables and fruits."

The native tribes located on the Pacific coast used to have parties called "potlatch" every time they had good luck in hunting this is because as a tradition they had to share the luck they had so no one would go without eating also it was a chance to have a party where they could have fun and who wouldn't want that even today? After several days when the guests left they would take away all the leftover food and use it for the return trip. These potlatch dinners have changed their name to pot luck for white people and they are nothing but frequent social gatherings in rural America. The meeting place is usually the parish hall or school cafeteria; the various dishes are placed on a table, and then tasted, compared and enjoyed by all.

Maple syrup is also a teaching of the American Indians that was passed on to the settlers who learned how to carve the bark to bring out the nectar at the right time of year. Corn and clam chowder are still the favorite soups in New England. Finally, it seems that two of our contemporary vices, gum and tobacco, also derive from American Indians, who were also drinkers. Some drank a light beer made from corn, potatoes, and peanuts; in certain months, along the East Coast, they drank a particular wine made from wild grapes. For the rest of the year, those tribes resorted to drinks obtained by boiling in water ginger, cinnamon, sassafras and other aromatic herbs. A recipe which seems to be very similar to certain "bubbly" beverages which today in the USA and all over the world are very popular!

Cooking Methods

Cooking in Buffalo Stomach

Before they met the white man, the Plains Indians cooked almost all of their food without utensils. Instead of metal pots, they used, for example, bison stomachs. This "pot" was also eaten. The washed stomach is hung on the tripod and inside water is poured and meat is added. Stones are heated on the fire and when they are hot they are put inside the stomach, when the first stone is immersed the water boils.

When the boiling calms down another stone is added.

Cooking under ground

Another way of cooking is under the ground. A pit is dug 60 cm deep and 60 cm wide. It is covered with stones and inside the fire is lit for about an hour, until the stones become hot. Once the fire is out, the embers are removed and the covering of hot stones is left in place. On the plains, the hole would be lined with a freshly tanned skin. Farther west, however, where trees grew, people lined the pit with tender green leaves of maple, sassafras, linden or wild vine. We tried using corn leaves. According to the directions, we lined the well with a layer of corn leaves, on which we placed the meat with the side dish (potatoes, corn, etc.). Today, as meat, chicken or smoked ham is fine. The more squeamish can wrap the meat in foil.

We cover it with another layer of leaves and close the hole with hot coals and earth. The "oven" is then left quiet for a few hours.

In the old days, the Indians prepared a large amount of grilled meat. The meat rested directly on the hot coals.

The best coals are obtained from hardwoods. In the absence of this type of wood, willow can be a good substitute.

Dried meat

The Indians did nothing for the future but prepare for winter. In the villages you could see racks everywhere with dried meat that could be made from any piece of meat.

They cut the meat following the natural contours and layers of muscle; they didn't cut it diagonally or saw through the bones like white people do. Dried meat has the advantage of being very light, nutritious and very good. Today, dried meat can be bought in supermarkets under the name of "jerky", however it does not have all the nutritional values as the Indian one which does not contain neither salts nor added additives.

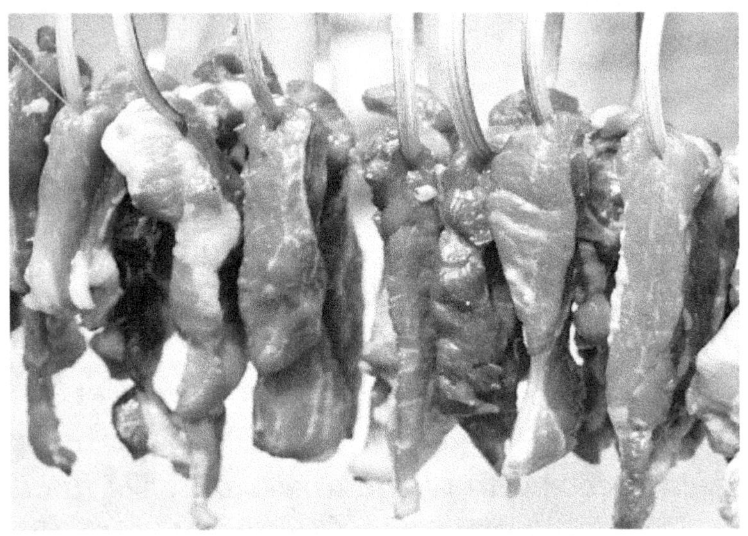

The Lakota made ba'pa (jerky in Lakota language) by drying strips of meat in the sun.

Making ba'pa requires a very sharp butcher knife. First, cut straight through the center of the piece of meat (about a pound in weight), stopping a few millimetres before completing the cut. Next, the process is to lay the meat first on one side then the other.

Do not be discouraged if the operation is very long. Sharp wooden skewers were used to hold the strips open during the drying process.

The strips were then hung on the poles of the dryers, high enough so that dogs could not steal the meat. Don't worry about the flies: the meat is only a few millimetres thick, so they cannot ruin it, as they cannot lay their eggs. The drying process lasts a few days.

During the night the meat should be laid on a cloth, in order to protect it from humidity. When it rains, the meat is hung on a string, inside the tepee. In this case it is smoked.

Pemmican

Pemmican is a mixture of ba'pa, dried cherries and fat. The dried meat is seared over the embers and then pounded in the mortar; to this are added the pounded cherries and bison fat. When everything is well mixed, egg-shaped patties are made. It is a very nutritious food, which was kept for the winter and periods when game was scarce.

Pemmican was eaten as is or used to make soup.

It was also used by the military and in the many polar expeditions. American soldiers, at that time, made exchanges with Indians in order to get it.

Even today, in the American army, a variant of the old pemmican is used.

Native American food recipes

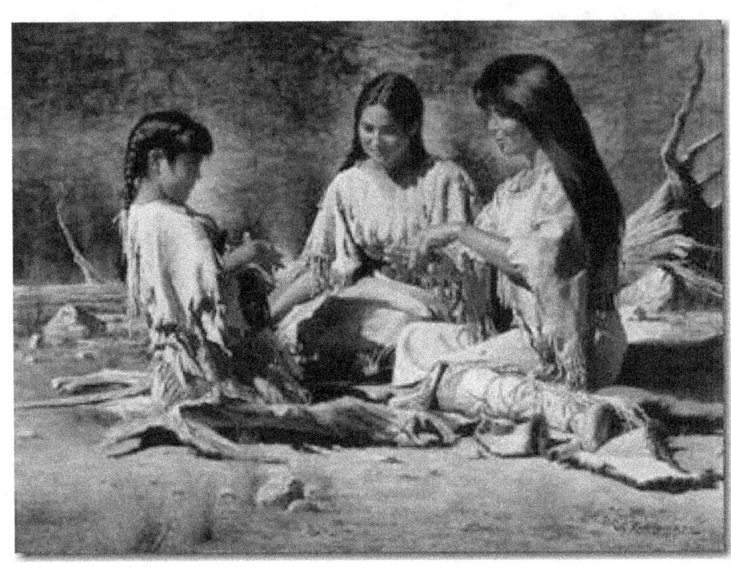

What follows is intended to be only a simplified list of the many recipes that the cultures of Native Americans adopted to survive with the little they could get and that ended up teaching the European pilgrims who arrived by ship from the continent, hence was created thanks giving or thanksgiving. Some of the recipes are placed here only for information because animals such as squirrels are not eaten by us while other animals may have laws that decline public consumption.

Trout soup

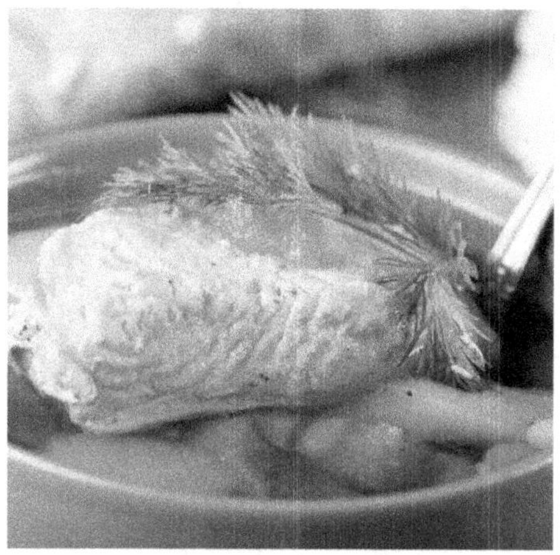

Preparation

Take 1 kg of trout, clean them, add a large potato cut into pieces, 1 white onion, 6 juniper berries, 300 gr. of spinach, 5 mint leaves, and a little water. Cook everything for about 20 minutes, then add a knob of butter; serve with chopped parsley and dill weed.

Tomato Soup

Ingredients:

- *1 kg tomatoes,*
- *3 potatoes cut into cubes*
- *one apple*
- *one white onion*
- *a pinch of fresh mint*
- *a tablespoon of sunflower oil,*
- *one tablespoon of oatmeal,*
- *5 leaves of fresh basil*
- *a tuft of dill weed,*
- *water as needed.*

Preparation:

Cook all ingredients for about two hours, minus the basil and dill, which should be added 10 minutes before the end of cooking.

Yellow pumpkin soup

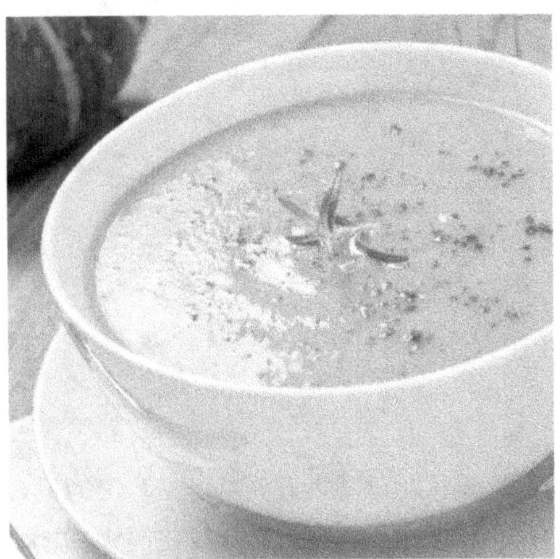

Preparation

Boil 1 kg of diced yellow pumpkin, 2 fresh spring onions thinly sliced, a tablespoon of honey, a tablespoon of sunflower oil, water to taste, a tuft of fresh dill. When cooked, purée the ingredients to obtain a puree, and garnish with the toasted sunflower seeds. Serve hot or cold.

Algonquin Walnut Soup (Paganenes)

Ingredients:

- 700 g crushed hazelnuts
- 6 shallots with tops
- 3 tablespoons chopped parsley
- 6 cups vegetable broth
- 1 teaspoon salt
- 1/4 teaspoon black pepper

Place all ingredients in a large pot and cook slowly
over medium heat for an hour and a half, stirring occasionally

Bell pepper soup - Cherokee

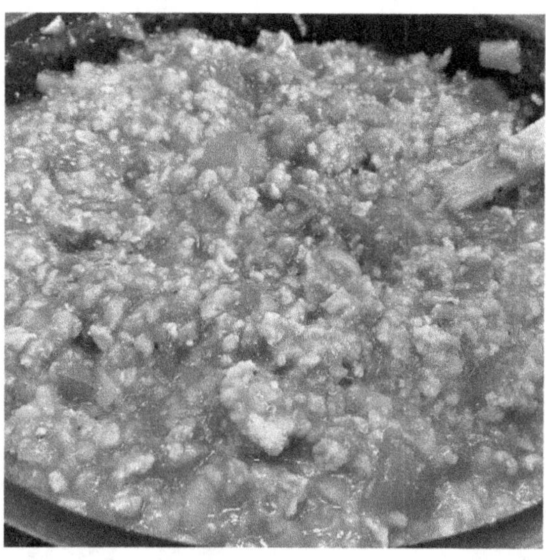

Ingredients:

- ½ kg beef or bone-in venison
- 2 l water
- 2 onions cut into quarters
- 2 tomatoes, seeded and diced
- 1 sweet bell pepper, seeded and diced
- 1 cup of okra, known by many names, including Bamia and Quingombo
- ½ cup diced potatoes
- ½ cup chopped carrot
- ½ cup corn
- 1/4 cup chopped celery
- salt, pepper

Place the meat, water, and onions in a heavy soup pot .

Cover and bring to a boil. Decrease heat to low and cook for 3 hours. Remove the meat, let it cool, remove the bones, and return it to the broth. Add the vegetables and simmer again, with a lid on halfway through, for an hour and a half. Season with salt and pepper.

Classic Chili

Ingredients:

- 1 kg of minced Beef meat (better if made with a knife),
- 600 gr. of cooked red beans,
- oil,
- 1 chopped onion,
- 1 chopped celery rib,
- 2 crushed garlic cloves,
- 2 level tablespoons of flour,
- 1 pinch of oregano,
- 1 tablespoon paprika,
- 1 teaspoon hot chili pepper,
- 1 pinch cumin powder, salt and pepper to taste.

Preparation:

Place the oil, onion and celery in a pot and brown; then add the meat and brown over high heat, stir in the flour and cook for another 2 minutes; then add the tomatoes,1/2 cup water and all other ingredients except the beans. Simmer for at least an hour, and then, add the beans, letting them season for another 20 minutes. Serve hot.

New potatoes with leeks

Preparation:

In a pan with a high rim, put 10 new potatoes (better if they are the same size), 3 large leeks, cleaned and chopped, a tablespoon of maple syrup, a nut, or meat concentrate, water as needed. Cook all ingredients together until cooked through and serve hot.

Succotash

Preparation:

Cook in a saucepan: one onion finely chopped, one green bell pepper chopped into pieces, 300 gr. of lima quality beans, 300 gr. of yellow corn, 2 tablespoons of nut butter, salt. At the end of cooking serve hot.

Succotash mohegan

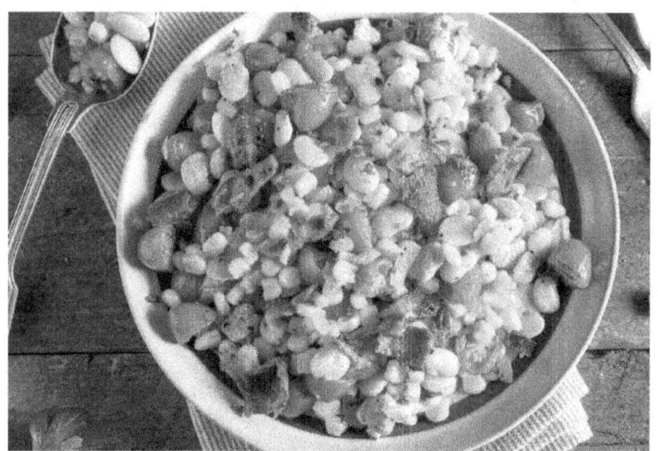

Ingredients:

- 1⁄2 cup sunflower oil,
- 2 medium white onions, chopped,
- 1 clove garlic,
- 2 chopped fresh spring onions,
- 2 ounces fresh wheat (grains),
- salt, pepper,
- 1 kg. lima beans,

- 1 zucchini, diced,
- 1 red bell pepper, 1 green bell pepper roasted and cut into strips,
- 3 cups chicken broth,
- 3 chopped fresh spring onions,
- 1 handful chopped parsley.

Preparation

Heat the oil in a small pan, add the onion and cook for one minute, then add the garlic and cook for another 5 minutes. Add pepper or paprika to taste, and stir. Top with the beans, corn, zucchini, and peppers, mixing well. To the ingredients, then add broth, just enough, and simmer 3 minutes over high heat, then lower the heat, and cook for about 15 minutes, when done, add the fresh spring onions and parsley and let stand for another 5 minutes with the heat off.

Roast Deer with wild rice

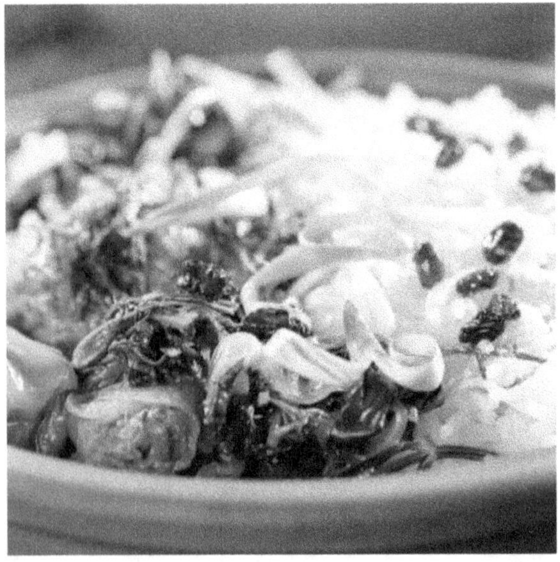

Take about 2 and 1/2 Kg. of venison, 5 or 6 juniper berries, salt then bind wrapping the meat with slices of bacon, oil, roast in the oven for about 1 and 1/2 hours at 180°, basting every now and then with a marinade prepared as follows: 2 glasses of apple vinegar, two tablespoons of honey or maple syrup, all heated to dissolve and mix the honey. Serve the meat in slices, over boiled wild rice.

Stewed rabbit with boiled dumplings (DUMPLINGS)

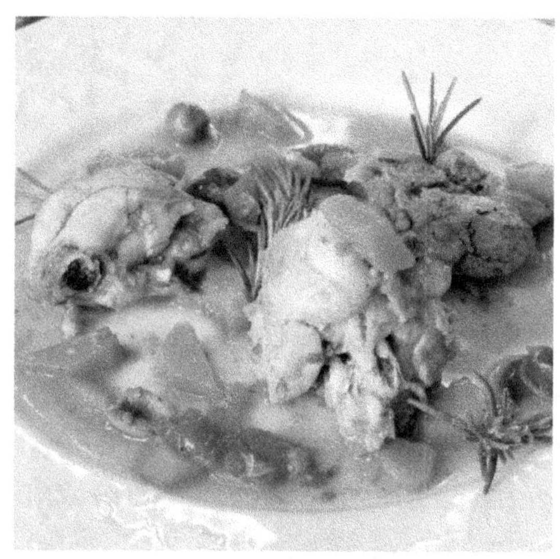

Clean and cut into pieces a rabbit weighing about 2 kg. Then dip each piece of meat in corn oil, and then in corn flour, brown in a pan, turning often, add about 1/2 litre of water and half a glass of apple vinegar, cook for about an hour after which, add 6 juniper berries, 8 small onions, 6 carrots into chunks, a tuft of dill weed and continue cooking for another 30 minutes. To make the DUMPLINGS take 2 ounces of oat flour, the egg, a tablespoon of nut butter and a glass of water. Mix all the ingredients well and throw the soft mixture (with the help of a spoon) into the rabbit sauce already made and cook for 10 minutes.

Partridge or duck with grapes and apples

Ingredients:

- One partridge or duck of about 2 1/2 kg,

- 250 gr. of sliced mushrooms,
- 3 hundred grams of grapes cut in half,
- 8 small potatoes whole,
- 3 chopped green apples
- 100 g. of peanuts,
- 6 small onions whole,
- 6 medium carrots in chunks,
- 2 cups apple vinegar,
- partridge entrails cleaned and chopped.

Preparation

Boil the entrails separately, then make a mixture by combining the mushrooms, grapes, apples, peanuts, juniper and a little salt. With the mixture obtained fill the partridge or duck, sew it up, place in a baking pan with the potatoes, carrots and onions and bake in the oven at 200° for about an hour, basting with apple vinegar diluted with a little water. After the first 20 minutes of cooking, reduce the temperature to 150°.

Quail with American peanuts

Ingredients:

- Choose 6 nice, plump quail,
- 2 ounces of oatmeal,
- sunflower oil,
- 3 tablespoons nut butter,
- 3 ounces of grapes,
- 100 grams of peanuts,
- two glasses of hot water,
- salt.

Preparation

Dip the quails in oil and then in flour. Melt the butter in a pan and cook the quails over medium heat, turning often, then add the water, grapes and continue cooking for about 40 minutes. Separately, toast the peanuts in the oven (for this, of course, remember to take the natural peanuts and not the salted ones already prepared) until golden brown, serve the quails with boiled rice and garnish with the peanuts.

Roast Turkey

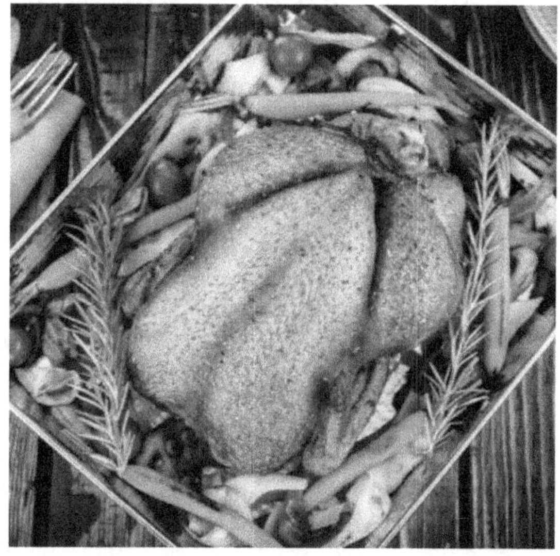

The turkey represents what is truly American besides tomatoes, peppers and corn: in the wild this bird was very difficult to hunt because it was agile and quick in getting up in flight, not like today when it is too big and cannot even fly anymore.

Recipe: clean a medium-sized turkey well, flaming it, rub it both inside and out with lemon, and stuff it with a filling of ground chestnuts, celery, bread crumbs, a teaspoon of thyme, one of marjoram and a pinch of chopped parsley, salt and pepper, oil. Sew up the opening of the turkey and place it in a baking pan, putting some sprigs of rosemary in the middle of the wings, and bake for about an hour at 170°, then sprinkle with white wine and continue cooking for another two and a half hours. Allow to cool before cutting.

Southern States Stew

The original preparation of this dish was made with the meat of the Squirrel, today it is replaced by the meat of Hare or Rabbit. Clean and cut in pieces a hare and boil it with an onion, when cooked drain it and bone it making small pieces, put in the broth already obtained 500 gr. of crushed tomatoes, 700 gr. of potatoes already boiled and cut in segments, 200 gr. of cooked broad beans, 300 gr. of corn in grains, salt and cayenne pepper. When the ingredients have taken on flavour, add them to the pieces of hare or rabbit, adding the broth, which will have become very creamy, and serve hot.

Mushroom Pie

Preparation:

Cook 3 fistfuls of field mushrooms (cleaned) in walnut butter until golden brown, separately prepare mashed potatoes with an egg in them and cover with this ,the bottom of a baking pan, add the mushrooms, a pinch of chopped parsley, a finely chopped spring onion and pulverize with a little oatmeal and fresh dill. Bake at 230° for about 25 minutes serve hot.

Crab fritters with chimichuri sauce

Ingredients:

- 3 ounces flaked crab,
- 5 whole eggs,
- 112 cup of chicken broth,
- corn oil,
- 1 chopped celery,
- 1 small white onion, chopped,

- *sunflower oil,*
- *2 ounces of yellow wheat flour,*
- *paprika,*
- *white pepper,*
- *finely chopped parsley and dill weed,*
- *lemon juice,*
- *salt.*

Preparation

In a frying pan heat the sunflower oil together with the onion, and cook for 1 minute, then add the parsley and a pinch of the yellow flour, cook for another 5 minutes, then remove and let cool. Then add all the other ingredients and allow to season for about 2 hours. Make pancakes and fry them in corn oil, letting them brown, drain and keep warm.

For the "chimichurri" sauce to add to the fritters, proceed as follows: take some chopped fresh parsley, some mint leaves, 1 large white onion finely chopped, 4 cloves of crushed garlic, 1 teaspoon of oregano, 1/2 glass of balsamic vinegar, 1/2 glass of red wine vinegar, black pepper, 1 small glass of olive oil. Mix all the ingredients together then let them rest for about 20 minutes, then sprinkle over the fritters and serve.

Shrimp Cajun style

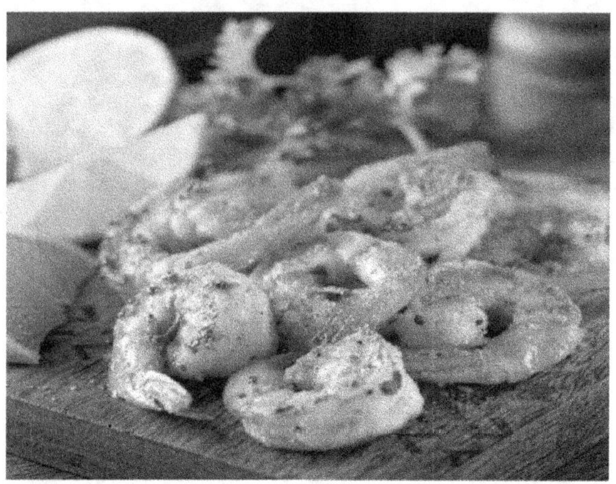

The Cajun Tribe calls shrimps, abundant in the area of the Gulf of Mexico, Crawfish, (dirty water shrimps) is their basic dish and the cooking of shrimps is done by drowning them in the cooking sauce. In a large saucepan, put some sunflower oil and add chopped onion, garlic, celery, when browned, add 100 gr. of flour by sprinkling and mix well. After a few minutes, add 400 gr. of shelled shrimps and let them brown, then pour in the pan 1/2 litre of vegetable broth, salt, cayenne pepper and cook for about 20 minutes. Generally these shrimps are served over boiled rice, still hot.

Navajo Fried Bread

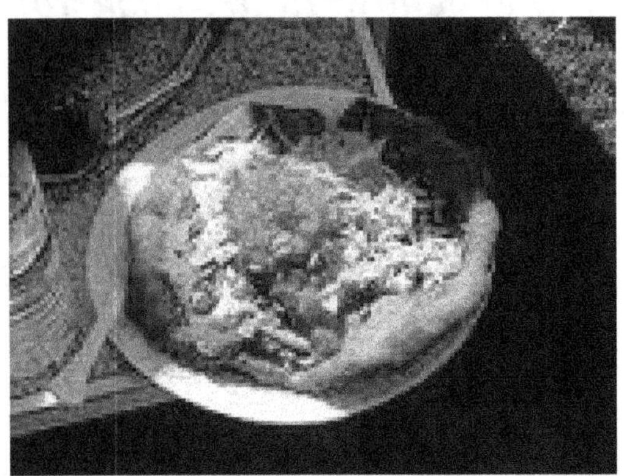

Ingredients:

- 3 ounces flour,
- 1/2 ounce ground sunflower seeds,
- 1 tablespoon baking powder,
- 2 tablespoons of oil.

Preparation

Mix all the ingredients together well, making a ball and leave to rest for about 2 hours. Then make round flattened rolls of about 1 cm. heat the oil and fry the rolls on both sides.

Bean Bread

Ingredients:

- 500 g beans;
- 750 g of yellow flour.

Preparation

Cook the beans in hot water. Sift the corn flour. Mix the beans with the flour, using the cooking water to make a soft dough. Form into loaves and bake in a hot oven until golden brown (you can also make sweet potato bread using the same process).

Indian Dumplings With Sauce

Ingredients:

- 3 cups cornmeal;
- one teaspoon of salt;
- 1 teaspoon baking soda.

Preparation

Mix ingredients well, pouring in boiling water until a firm dough is obtained. Cut out small balls and cook them in boiling salted water for 15 minutes. For the sauce, take two tablespoons of the batter, dilute it until it becomes a creamy consistency and cook it for 20 minutes.

Battered Pumpkin Flowers

Ingredients:

- 2 to 3 dozen squash blossoms (preferably unopened);
- 1 cup milk;
- ½ cup oil for frying;
- 1 tablespoon flour;

- *pepper;*
- *salt;*
- *paprika.*

Preparation

Mix together the flour, milk, salt and pepper. Invert the mixture over the squash blossoms arranged in an ovenproof dish. Heat the oil and fry the flowers until golden brown. Pat dry with paper towels and sprinkle with paprika before serving.

Indian Mohawk Corn

Ingredients:

- *1 can corn;*
- *nuts;*
- *butter.*

Preparation

Pour 1 can of corn into a pot, add butter and chopped walnuts. Add water and cook. Serve hot.

Baked Cucumbers

Ingredients:

- *4 cucumbers, peeled and cut into four pieces lengthwise;*
- *1 tablespoon crushed dill seeds;*
- *2 tablespoons butter or margarine;*
- *pepper and salt.*

Preparation

Arrange a layer of cucumbers in the bottom of an ovenproof dish and spread with half of the butter or margarine. Mix together the spices and sprinkle half of them over the cucumbers. Add a second layer and top with the rest of the butter and spices. Bake in a 350 degree oven for 45 minutes (halfway through baking, gently turn cucumbers over to brown evenly on both sides). Serve piping hot.

Cherokee Bean Patties

Ingredients:

- 2 cups black beans;
- 4 cups cornmeal;
- ½ cup white flour;
- 1 teaspoon baking soda.

Preparation

Boil beans in water until tender. Pour cornmeal, flour and baking soda into a large mixing bowl and mix thoroughly. Add the boiling beans, along with a little of the cooking water, to form a firm dough. Cut out small balls, to be cooked for 30 minutes over low heat in boiling water.

Chippewa fritters

Ingredients:

- 3 ounces oatmeal,
- 1/2 litre water,
- 1/2 glass of oil,
- 1/2 glass of liquid honey,
- oil for frying.

Preparation

Mix all the ingredients together well and add the honey last, then heat the oil in a pan and fry the mixture in spoonfuls, when the fritters are golden brown on both sides put them to drain on absorbent paper and serve immediately hot.

American Walnut and Pumpkin Pie

Ingredients:

- 2 ounces oat flour (fine type),
- 2/3 cup potato flour,
- 2/3 cup pumpkin (cooked),
- 2/3 cup chopped walnuts,
- 1 egg,
- 1/2 glass of maple syrup.

Preparation

Mix the flours and slowly amalgamate the other ingredients, making a homogeneous dough, then pour it into an oiled baking pan and bake at 180° for about 1 hour.

Baked Pumpkin

Ingredients:

- 1 small pumpkin;
- 2 tablespoons cider or apple juice;
- 2 tablespoons honey;
- 2 tablespoons melted butter or margarine.

Preparation

Wash the pumpkin thoroughly, arrange it whole in an ovenproof dish and bake it for 1 1/2 hours at 350°. Take it out of the oven and make a hole on the top in order to extract the seeds. Mix together the honey, cider and margarine and pour into the pumpkin. Cover and bake again for 30 minutes, adding more cider sauce from time to time to keep it from drying out. Serve at the table whole or in slices.

Hazelnut Cookies

Ingredients:

- 300 gm ground dry hazelnuts,
- 2 ounces oat flour (fine type),
- 1 teaspoon of maple syrup,
- 2 cups water,
- oil for frying.

Preparation

Boil the nuts in water for about half an hour, then add the syrup and oatmeal, mix well and let stand until thickened. Prepare a pan with hot oil and cook the mixture in spoonfuls on both sides. The resulting cookies are served either hot or cold in place of bread.

Sweet Potato Treats

Ingredients:

- 4 large sweet potatoes;
- 3 eggs;
- 1 teaspoon salt;
- a pinch of pepper;
- oil for frying.

Preparation

Boil potatoes until tender, peel and mash. Add the eggs, salt and pepper. Heat the oil and fry the mixture by spoonfuls until golden brown, creating small flattened discs with the help of a spatula. Serve warm with butter and honey.

Sunflower seed cake

Ingredients:

- 3 ounces sunflower seeds,
- dry or fresh,
- 1/2 lt water,
- oatmeal,
- 2 teaspoons of maple syrup,
- 1/2 glass of oil.

Preparation

Cook the sunflower seeds in the water, then drain and marinate by combining the oatmeal and maple syrup, making a fairly thick paste. With this, form small cakes and brown them in hot oil on both sides.

CONCLUSION

Thank you for making it to the end of this book, we hope it has been informative and able to provide you with all the tools you need to achieve your goals, whatever they may be.

This book is here to help you improve both your physical and spiritual well-being.

As you continue your journey, keep this book close by for reference and inspiration.

Make sure you are not hurting others, in your words and actions. Strive to live in harmony with nature by making sure you do not upset the ecological balance.

All you have to do is embrace the tools, use your intuition, let nature be your guide and open yourself up to the possibilities of everything around you in the natural world.

Walking the Native American path is a devotion to yourself and to the elements of Earth and nature.

I hope this book can help you achieve your goals.

Finally, if you found this book helpful in any way, a review on Amazon is always appreciated!

www.ingramcontent.com/pod-product-compliance
Lightning Source LLC
Chambersburg PA
CBHW080443030726
47592CB00011B/2943